#MS

Imprint

1ˢᵗ Edition
October 2024
Jasminka Vuković 10000 Zagreb, Croatia
Coauthor: Mia Madalena Vuković
Cover design: Studio Lingua d.o.o., Zagreb, Croatia
Editor: Studio Lingua d.o.o., www.studio-lingua.hr
Layout designer: Joh.-Chr. Hanke
Copyright ©2024 by Jasminka Vuković
info@studio-lingua.hr

Jasminka Vuković

#MS—We'll get rid of it

An autobiographical novel

Book
Mother and daughter, friends and allies for life. Her nineteen-year-old daughter Mia is studying veterinary medicine when she suddenly finds herself unable to hold the scalpel any longer. The initial diagnosis? Just normal stress symptoms. But three years later, frightening symptoms reappear, and an examination in the emergency room reveals shocking results. The final diagnosis: incurable Multiple Sclerosis. At first, Mia seems to manage just fine, juggling university, social media hashtags, and a trip to London. When she then falls in love with sports student Ben, her happiness appears perfect. Yet... something in this relationship takes a wrong turn. Shortly after, Mia's condition deteriorates—also because a super medication shows no effect.

Mia becomes a case requiring constant care.

How does Ben react? What does daily life look like for daughter and mother, suddenly navigating a world of wheelchairs, hospital gloom, and catheters? And what if the doctors' prognoses are wrong, and Mia holds a secret key to reclaiming her vibrant life?

A story of unconditional love. Of hope that demands true determination. And of days when happiness is just a heartbeat away.

For my daughter Mia Madalena, the light of my life

– Chapter 1 –

Tuesday, February 2, 2016

"That makes seventy-five dollars. Unfortunately, we only accept cash," the receptionist explains with a smile.

"Do you happen to have a calming pill for me? It's nothing serious, right? Surely it can be treated, can't it?" With trembling fingers, I put the money on the reception desk.

"Yeah, sure," she responds in a tone that is obviously meant to reassure me. Then she hands me a pill. She continues to smile and gestures with her head towards the water container in the empty waiting room. She just wants me to pay and leave, I think, not knowing whether I should be annoyed or surprised.

Meanwhile, Mia and Tony are standing behind me at the reception desk, appearing impatient. I can tell from the looks on their faces that they don't know what to make of all this either.

"What did she say?" Tony asks me quietly, looking first at me and then at the receptionist. It seems like he's trying to gauge the seriousness of the situation from her expression.

"I don't know. We have to go for an emergency CT scan at the hospital. To the emergency room. 'Right away', she said," I reply, struggling to maintain composure.

Everything will be okay, I repeat in my mind, trying not to spill the water in the plastic cup. Everything will be okay. Words that are meant to calm me down. But I feel nauseous and my pulse is racing.

Five minutes later, we leave the private practice and get into the car with the neurologist's findings.

At exactly two o'clock, we reach the emergency room. My ears are ringing and the bright fluorescent lighting in treatment room number 7 is almost unbearable. Only a half-open glass door separates the room from the corridor, through which a man shouts that he is in pain. Nurses and doctors hurry back and forth in the emergency room corridor. The pungent smell of disinfectant hangs everywhere in the heated air.

My heart is racing wildly as we stand indecisively in the tiny treatment room, waiting to see the doctor. I feel like I could faint at any moment. What are we doing here, I ask myself.

"Well, there's nothing abnormal on the CT scan," the doctor's voice suddenly reaches me from the door.

I sit down on a chair and start to cry. So it's just from stress after all, I think with relief. Tony puts a comforting hand on my shoulder.

"When did she start having these symptoms?" the doctor asks, turning to me.

"The numbness started in one arm a few days ago. Then it went on and on, spreading to other areas. On Sunday, the skin on my stomach suddenly went completely numb. I noticed it in bed in the morning. Now I feel like I have a tight corset around my waist," Mia replies.

She sits down next to me and tries to take a deep breath. As if she wants to demonstrate to the doctor what she means by the corset.

"The neurologist said I could just be imagining it. The numbness. Or it could be from the stress at university. As if I would make up something like this. I have nothing better to do than sit here in the emergency room," she explains, rolling her eyes.

"You should get an MRI of the brain. That way, we can see if everything is okay with the central nervous system," the doctor explains, staring at the report.

That sounds plausible, I think. Just check everything, and then we'll have proof that it's just stress anyway. No wonder, with all those exams at the university. Especially now that she no longer lives at home.

Meanwhile, two months must have passed since Mia moved to the other end of the city to live in a small apartment with a fellow student. She wanted to experience what it's like to live alone. Being independent, not having to sign in and out at home, as she puts it.

I'm aware that this way she can also meet her boyfriend Josh whenever she wants. Without Mom knowing when she's coming home. At twenty-one, that's understandable.

In my confusion of thoughts, suddenly, an actress comes to mind. One side of her face was paralyzed from one day to the next. Due to stress. Or was it a TV host? She's recovered too. The other day in the magazine she looked completely normal and happy again. Stress can really take a toll. And having the central nervous system checked sounds like we've thoroughly examined everything.

"It's best if you have this done privately," the doctor snaps me out of my thoughts. "You can get an appointment more quickly at a private clinic, and I'd like to see the findings next week." He sits down at the computer and types the report in silence, the minutes stretching into eternity.

"Today is Tuesday. Mia, please come next Monday to the Neurology Day Clinic with the report. Green building, fourth floor. Make sure you have a referral from your general practitioner. We'll reassess from there," he explains to her. "Please get an appointment from the nurse."

He hands the report to the young nurse at the door and leaves treatment room number 7 with a nod in our direction.

Doctor Richards, neurologist I read later at the very bottom right of the report.

"We still have an available MRI appointment on Friday. Would 3 p.m. be okay for you?" enthusiastically says a lady from the Radiology Clinic, an hour later, over the phone.

Pleasant receptionist, I think, picturing her balancing the phone between her ear and shoulder while typing the appointment into the computer. A pleasant voice. Everything is pleasant, I think, only the reason for my call is not pleasant.

"Yes, that's okay. Is there anything to keep in mind? Does she need to fast or anything?"

"No, that's not necessary," she responds. "Just bring your daughter's medical records."

Alright, so it's Friday, I repeat in my mind, jotting down the appointment in my desk calendar. That's two and a half more days to go.

Days during which I place the report from the emergency room in the hallway on our wooden chest of drawers, attempting to ignore it. Or rather, trying to ignore it. Because I'm aware that it must contain a suspected diagnosis. A suspicion that I neither want to see nor know about. Out of fear of what it might mean.

Meanwhile, Mia is back at her place with her fellow student in their shared apartment. That's what she wanted. She feels good enough, she says, and it distracts her.

Around six o'clock, Tony and I silently have dinner—leftovers. He looks at me repeatedly, offering a comforting smile. A smile that is meant to console me. One that says, 'Everything will be fine. I am here.' I smile back. More to reassure myself that this will have a positive outcome, and I am worrying unnecessarily.

When I feel the first signs of an impending migraine an hour later, I decide to remove my makeup and go to bed. Preferably with a sleeping pill.

Wednesday, February 3

On Wednesday morning, I wake up at six. I've hardly slept last night. I had constant nightmares about receiving calls from the hospital. CT machines pulling Mia into a tube and not spitting her out.

Spending the day mostly in front of the TV on the couch, I pretend to watch some series in silence. In between, I call Mia repeatedly under different pretenses. Then, I ask her casually if the numbness might have subsided.

No, she confirms repeatedly what I don't want to hear. In the evening, she goes to a café with her fellow student, and there's no need for me to call her again. I shouldn't worry, she says. We'll talk tomorrow.

Meanwhile, the report still lies on the chest of drawers in the hallway. I keep catching a brief glance of it out of the corner of my eye as I walk past. *Encephalitis*, I think I read. I feel nauseous again.

Remind yourself what that could mean, I admonish myself. After all, you've translated hundreds of medical reports. You know these medical terms.

It's probably meningitis, it occurs to me. Shouldn't that be treated immediately? Why didn't the doctor provide clear information? I did ask him. Maybe I should Google it now. No, I'd better not, I think the next moment. Because then I won't make it through the days until the appointment on Friday.

In the end, I put a magazine on the report to cover it. Now, as I pass by, I can't read what might be written in the report. I'll find out on Friday anyway. Until then, I'll pretend like nothing happened. As if the world is in order, and nothing has changed.

So the day passes without me taking any notice of it, and by around four in the afternoon, it's already dark outside. I realize I've hardly eaten anything today as I sit in front of the TV in the evening. I stare at the screen, not really knowing what's on. Tony has fallen asleep on the couch and is snoring. Well, he's not her father, comes to my mind. But I do him injustice with this thought. He's played the role of a father in her life since she was nine. And he does it as well as any biological father could. I smile as I look at him, lying there so peacefully.

Then, just before midnight, I think I almost made it through Wednesday as I glance at the clock. Now, I just have to get through the sleeping part, and it will already be Thursday.

Thursday, February 4

Actually, I should be working on this Thursday morning. There are still several translations waiting for me on the desk. But I just can't. I feel paralyzed with fear of what could come tomorrow. That's why I decline client calls. I can't bear them right now. And I only briefly skim through incoming emails as well. Everything can wait because terrible thoughts constantly swirl in my head, and I can't focus on anything else. I can't stop thinking about what this examination and an MRI might reveal.

A vague sensation lingers with me all day, as if my body no longer obeys me properly. Tony tiptoes around me, as if he doesn't want to unnecessarily disturb me with his presence. Meanwhile, I repeatedly try to calm myself, convincing myself that if it were something serious, the doctor would have said something. He would have kept her in the hospital. He would have ordered an emergency surgery or something like that.

None of that happened, though. She was allowed to go home. Then it can't be that serious. On the other hand, he wants to see an MRI of her brain. What does he think he'll find with this MRI, I wonder. Everything was clearly visible on the CT. Namely, nothing. Nothing abnormal. No malignant tumor, no blood clots. Everything okay, he said.

But there was that look in his eyes. That evasiveness. As if he knew something more, something he doesn't want to say.

I've been thinking about that all day. While cooking, doing laundry, eating, and watching TV in the evening. About that look.

Friday, February 5

In half an hour, we have to leave. No matter how much I wished Friday were still far away, it's here. Mia is waiting for Tony and me at a bus stop halfway between the university and the Radiology Clinic at around two o'clock in the afternoon. We pick her up in the car.

She is doing well, she says as she gets in, claiming to have slept quite well.

"Just a little tired from the lectures," she explains with a smile.

I reach my arm back and gently stroke her knee. She smiles reassuringly. As if it were about me, not her.

Then Tony turns on the radio. This way, we can stay silent and don't have to talk about the upcoming examination. And I can observe her closely in the rearview mirror as we drive.

She's wearing makeup, has styled her long golden-brown hair. I imagine her curling each strand with a curling iron in the morning.

At the university, she surely attracts many glances, it occurs to me, and I have to smile. She looks good, not pale or sick. Just good, as always. And that eases my mind.

Shortly before three o'clock, Mia and I are sitting in a waiting area outside the MRI examination rooms. Tony paces impatiently up and down the corridor, and time seems to drag on.

"Are you nervous?" I ask Mia.

"No, not really. I just hope it doesn't take too long. You have to lie still and not move," she replies.

She seems calm, I think, as I observe her anxiously from the side. I, on the other hand, don't know where to channel my anxiety. I feel hot, and it seems like I can't stand the wait any longer. We sit quietly for a while in silence. Outwardly, I appear composed, I think, but deep down, I'd rather get up and walk away.

In my mind, I am five again, and it's Monday morning at six o'clock, and I have to go to the backup kindergarten because the summer vacation has already started, and my regular kindergarten is closed. My father tries to comfort me lovingly as he hands me over to a teacher at the kindergarten door. "Later, when Dad picks you up, we'll count the birds' nests in the trees again," he promises, embracing me tightly. But nothing can console me right now because I don't know the kids here, and I'll spend the whole day alone in the play corner. The entire long day with a stomachache and a longing for home.

Suddenly, a female voice pulls me out of my memories. Mia is called into the MRI treatment room. Tony and I can wait, explains the blonde receptionist and tells Mia to take off her jacket and handbag in a tiny changing room. She should also remove any jewelry, if she has any. It will take about half an hour, she explains to me.

That's a long time, I think, very long. But somehow, I have to sit here patiently until the time is over. Meanwhile, Tony sits beside me and gently strokes my hand. He knows I don't want to talk when I'm anxious, so he stays silent. It's his way of saying, "It will be okay. Don't worry."

However, a question weighs on my mind. So I approach one of the passing receptionists in the hallway.

"Excuse me. How long do we usually have to wait for the results? Are they sent by email, or do you call?"

She smiles kindly. "The doctor immediately reviews the MRI images on the CD and writes the report right after. Then you go into his treatment room and he explains what's visible in the images," she quickly explains and then rushes along the hallway.

"Good," I say, turning to Tony. "Then we'll know it today. I prefer that as well, rather than having to wait for days."

But I don't know if I really prefer that. Maybe I need a little more time. Time to get used to what's about to happen. To be able to pretend for just one or two more days that our life is still the same.

However, forty-five minutes later, an older doctor asks Mia, Tony and me into his treatment room. Only the light from the two computer screens illuminates the tiny room. He sits down behind his desk and gestures towards the chairs on the opposite wall. So we sit down, and I observe the doctor's facial expression, as if I could read something from it before he speaks. He stares thoughtfully at one of the screens and furrows his brow.

"You're the patient?" he asks, addressing Mia.

"Yes," she replies.

"Tell me, how long have you had these symptoms?" he asks, and I notice a slight hesitation in his voice.

"I've had this numbness for about two weeks now."

"And were there any other symptoms? Such as headaches, vision problems?"

"I've had headaches a lot in recent years. More like migraines. And in January, I got myself a new pair of glasses because I sometimes see things a bit blurry. I also had to change my major. Because of the trembling in my hands. I studied veterinary medicine and couldn't participate in practical exercises anymore—holding a scalpel, filling liquids into test tubes, and such."

"What are you studying now?" The doctor is obviously interested in Mia's future career and leans back in his office chair.

"PR and Media Studies. It wasn't my first choice, but what can I do?" Mia answers, looking over at me questioningly.

"Is there anything noticeable on the images?" I impatiently interject. What's the point of asking, I think annoyed.

"If you'd like to take a look here," he responds, pointing with a pen at one of the computer screens. The MRI image of a brain is visible on it. That of my daughter.

"Look, these small gray spots are chronic inflammations. And this large white area is an acute inflammation that triggers certain symptoms. Such as sensory disturbances, visual impairments, tremors, or the like."

Then it slowly dawns on me. This is one of those ›fatal car accident‹ situations. Two police officers stand in front of the relatives' door. The wife opens the door with a surprised look. She stands unknowingly in her kitchen apron in front of the officers, behind her a curious-looking toddler. The TV is on in the background. She's probably just preparing lunch and waiting for her husband.

"Ms. Lewis?" one of the police officers asks politely.

"Yes," she replies, more in question.

"May we come in?"

"Yes, of course." She steps aside so the officers can enter the house.

"There was a car accident on the highway. Your husband's vehicle was hit by another vehicle. He suffered severe injuries. And…"

The woman widens her eyes in horror, covers her mouth with her hands. She tries to suppress a stifled sob.

"We unfortunately have to inform you that he succumbed to his injuries."

In a matter of seconds, I'm back in the present, hearing myself asking: "And what do you think these inflammations mean? What could this be?"

He hesitates for a moment, biting his lip.

"Multiple sclerosis," he responds, strained, without meeting my gaze.

What does he mean by that? It can't be, I think, feeling my heart race suddenly. Mia is only twenty-one. It just can't be. My head is buzzing, and I feel dizzy. He's mistaken, he must be. I look at Mia. She sits quietly beside me. Her gaze doesn't even tell me what she's thinking. The disease has to go away. Somehow it has to go away, I think, confused.

"Are you sure?" I ask, almost in a panic, looking over at Tony.

"Pretty sure. There are only a few diseases with such lesions on the brain. The images are clear."

I sit rigid in my chair, but I want to scream. I want to shake the doctor. Want to beg him to change his mind. To name a less severe diagnosis as a possibility. A sudden realization hits me. Wheelchair. MS means a wheelchair. No, that simply cannot and should not be, I think in the next moment, horrified by this realization.

"I understand that this is difficult for you," the doctor begins calmly, looking first at Mia, then Tony and me. "But I have many patients who are doing very well. Just a few days ago, I had a sixty-seven-year-old gentleman who thought he had a chronic inflammation of the optic nerve for years. However, it turned out to be multiple sclerosis. So far, he's living wonderfully with it. Some even run marathons. One of my patients is a mountain climber and a high-performance athlete. He's doing great too."

Great, I think, then we should be happy that she was diagnosed in her early twenties and not in her late sixties. His words make me angry, but at the same time I draw some hope from it. Maybe it's not that bad after all. There must be gradations. From very mild MS to very severe, it comes to my mind.

However, this brief sense of relief, thinking it could only be a harmless variant for Mia, quickly fades, and fear takes hold within me. Because I realize that MS simply means MS and that the first symptoms have already become apparent. And all of this at her young age of twenty-one.

"It would be best if you show the images to your neurologist and seek advice," he says encouragingly, as if it were a common cold, and then stands up. That's probably the end of the patient consultation, I think, and we leave the treatment room.

On the parking lot in front of the Radiology Clinic, I stop in front of the car before we get in. I hug Mia silently. I can't even cry, the shock is too deep. My child, my only child, keeps echoing in my mind.

She feels nauseous, she says, and needs to sit in the back seat. Tony helps her to sit down but doesn't get in himself. I sit next to her in the car and hug her tightly to me.

"We'll get through this," I whisper, pressing my face against hers while struggling with tears. "Nowadays, there are certainly good treatment methods. There's always research being done. They have something against it. I'm sure of that."

But she stays silent and looks out the window as Tony starts driving.

"Are you coming home with us?" I ask her shortly after.

"It's still light outside, we could go for a coffee." So we don't have to go home, where there's time to think, I silently add in my thoughts.

She prefers to go to Josh and go out to distract herself, she replies. Actually, I would actually prefer to have her with me now. I want to lie down beside her in bed in the evening and hold her close. Never let her go again. Cry together with her. But she knows me, I think then. She can't bear my bewilderment right now.

After about twenty minutes of driving through the city, Tony stops at a bus stop to let Mia out of the car.

"You know, Mom, this might sound strange now, but somehow it's also a relief. Finally, all of this has a name. These strange symptoms over the years that no one could categorize. At last I'm not seen as a hypochondriac anymore," she says before getting out of the car.

And somehow she's right. Now all the symptoms of the last few years at least have a name. Though a frightening one.

Around eleven o'clock in the evening, I go to bed alone. The TV is on in the living room. Too loud, but it doesn't bother me tonight. Because the TV noises give me a sense of familiarity, and that comforts me. Earlier, before I went to brush my teeth,

I said to Tony that I wanted to read a bit to distract myself. He could go ahead and watch TV.

And now I'm lying here. Alone with my thoughts. A thriller lies on my nightstand, one I've been reading since last week. Or rather, used to read. In another life, I think sadly. The life where I comfortably curl up in bed with a book, the familiar routine of reading. Because it's part of my daily routine. Reading. It belongs to my normal world. That's where I want to go back. Simply close my eyes and return to the time before this nightmare began. But something has taken hold in my chest. Something heavy and painful. A realization, a knowledge of what could come in the future.

When I then glance at a photo on the opposite bedroom wall, pain tightens my throat. It shows me at the age of twenty-one. I'm holding my one-year-old daughter in my arms. The sea in the background. We are inseparable. Have always been. Like peas in a pod, Tony often jokes. At the thought of it, I start to cry. For the first time since this whole nightmare began. Fortunately, my father doesn't have to witness this anymore. That would have been too much for him, I think, while sobbing at the photo. Our little sweetie. My princess.

Why her and not me, I ask myself again and again. I have already lived my youth. I traveled, turned my passion into a profession. I found the right partner. What did I miss? I always tried to protect her. At twenty, I was young, I think as I look at myself in the photo. Moreover, a single parent, but that didn't stop me from being a good mother to her. I always wanted to prove to everyone: Look, I'm young, but I manage everything. My child is happy, I have a great job. I've built a career, I've climbed the ladder. Today, I'm my own boss.

Well, she was often sick when she was little, I remember. But who wasn't? Little ones constantly bring something from the kindergarten—infections, lice. Could I have done something about it? Were there warning signs I didn't recognize?

And what about all her complaints in recent years? She even

had to change her beloved course of study. Due to the intense trembling in her hands. Her colleagues at university noticed it at some point during the anatomy lectures, she told me at home one evening. She blamed it on hunger, saying to them she hadn't had breakfast.

But then she couldn't get away with it any more. It all came to a halt during a demonstration on the thigh of an animal cadaver. She cut her index finger with the scalpel because she simply couldn't hold it anymore, she later sobbed.

"Red meat, red berries," our family doctor, Doctor Field, advised her then. It was the stress that comes with such a demanding course of study, she explained. It was all just from stress. The constant headaches, the numbness in the hand at fourteen. It was attributed to playing the guitar, said the neurologist who, years later, would refer us for an emergency CT scan.

Then came the vision problems in January, the pain in her left leg. We haven't skipped any medical examination to find out where all of this is coming from. For years, I dragged her everywhere. From scintigraphy to EMNG to MRI of the spine. We visited neurologists and psychologists.

My friend Anne, a child and adolescent psychiatrist, finally suggested antidepressants. Antidepressants at that age, I didn't want that. At fifteen, you shouldn't take such things. After some deliberation, we reluctantly followed our friend Anne's advice.

When the antidepressants failed to help, and at the start of her studies, she developed an aversion to clothing on her skin, we knew we needed a different approach. I found a private psychotherapist for her. Conversations help, I thought naively at the time. But it didn't get any better.

Far Eastern medicine could be a solution, we then decided. She began regularly attending acupuncture sessions with a genuine Asian practitioner. Not a trained European. A real expert, I thought, who knows how to do this. When the sensory disturbances and the constant migraine-like headaches worsened, we turned to homeopathy.

"Stretch your arms forward. Palms facing down. Place a vial of various globules under each palm, and then we'll see which ones suit you," the homeopath instructed Mia.

Well, I thought. That's settled now. From now on, she'll take globules. Unfortunately, that didn't work either. And it was expensive, too. Like all the other attempts at treatment. And did it help in any way? No, I think bitterly.

Now we're left with a diagnosis that I never expected in a thousand years. How can it be that not a single doctor came up with the idea of assigning the individual symptoms to a specific illness, I ask myself, feeling a mix of sorrow and something akin to anger. Our family doctor, Doctor Field, should have had some inkling.

I feel like screaming out loud. But instead, I start to pray. I pray to all the known entities of the Catholic heavenly realm. At first, my prayers are humble and pleading, but soon they turn desperate and demanding. God, Mary and Jesus should fix it. Who else can help me now, I ask aloud, tears streaming down my face as I gaze at the image of Mary on the opposite bedroom wall. You must know the answers. You are omniscient. Then help me.

Then I turn to the universe. I close my eyes and try to formulate a clear wish in my mind. As I have often read and tried. The law of attraction and such. A sense of embarrassment washes over me, mingled with the desperation of my plea. It feels foolish and futile, yet I cling to it with desperate hope. From God to the Universe. Everything seems acceptable to me at this moment. We just have to get rid of this disease. No matter how.

As tiredness finally overwhelms me, my mother comes to mind in the semi-consciousness of sleep. Tomorrow I still have the phone call with her ahead. But how do you tell your own mother that her grandchild is incurably ill?

A week later, we arrive at the Neurology Day Clinic at seven in the morning. Doctor Richards has ordered a lumbar puncture after we presented him with the MRI findings at the agreed-upon appointment last Monday. The puncture is necessary for us to have final clarity, as brain lesions can occur in some other conditions, he explained.

So, I accompany Mia into the still empty treatment room of the day clinic, where Doctor Richards and three nurses are already waiting for us. It's cool in here, I notice right away. Probably the heating was just turned on. After all, Mia seems to be the first patient this morning.

One of the nurses briefly explains that I'm allowed to stay in the room during the puncture. However, I have to sit in a chair by the window, a bit away from the action.

Mia is asked to sit on one of the hospital beds. After a short preparation with a sterile cover on her back and other utensils that I'd rather not see, the procedure begins.

"Now, Mia, bend forward as far as you can. You'll feel a little prick in your spine soon, and it could be uncomfortable for a moment. Stay very still so nothing slips, and it won't take long. After it's all done, you can lie down for a bit," Doctor Richards explains to her as he performs the lumbar puncture.

"It's like an epidural anesthesia. A needle is inserted between the vertebrae in the back," I explained to Mia yesterday. "I had that during your birth when the labor pains became unbearable."

Only, in my daughter's case, cerebrospinal fluid is being extracted, I think sadly now, turning my gaze away so I don't have to see what is happening to Mia.

As I look out the window, I suddenly smile because I recall Mia's detailed explanation of the upcoming lumbar puncture earlier this morning on the way to the clinic. She had watched everything vividly and in color in a well-presented video on the internet. How can she? I asked myself. And the next moment, I thought: Well, her love for medicine.

However, when she began to create more images from the video in my mind, I'd had enough. Tony and I didn't want to know every detail, I explained to her. Besides, Tony should focus on driving.

Thinking about it makes me smile again, as about twenty minutes later, the puncture is finished. Mia has come through it well, Doctor Richards explains. It may take about ten days for the results to come in.

And his words are like a stab in the heart. Because I know that waiting this time will be a real test for me. These will be days I have to face alone. Without Tony, who has to travel for his construction company. And without Mia, who returns to her shared apartment tomorrow.

So, the upcoming days drag on slowly and seem to pull me along like a current. From morning to evening. And then to the next day. Each day follows the same pattern. I wake up around seven o'clock and spend the rest of the day mostly on my laptop or quietly wandering through the apartment. Wrapped in my warm bathrobe. Despite the heating, I struggle against a persistent cold that seems to have penetrated every fiber of my body. I can't bear this cold and silence. That's why the television runs in the background from morning until night.

In these days, my daily routine revolves around the clinic's office hours. From eight in the morning to three in the evening. During this time, Doctor Richards could call me to share the results of the lumbar puncture.

That's why I don't eat anything until three o'clock and constantly check the clock. On the laptop screen, in the living room, in the kitchen. A glance from the corner of my eye, a brief look, or a direct check of how much time is left until the end of the office hours. Hoping for the call on one hand. On the other hand, silently pleading for some delay. Secretly, I picture a miracle, an outcome even the doctors didn't expect.

›Well, we've never had this before. It's not MS; it's just inflammations that we can quickly get rid of. A bit of antibiotics, and the issue will be resolved.‹

But these are probably just wishful scenarios.

In between, I attempt to work, although I would prefer to crawl into bed and cry. Unfortunately, my translation agency doesn't allow for that. As the company CEO, you don't lie down and cry. You're tough, I bitterly think, no matter how life unfolds. At least I work from home, it then comes to my mind. Given my current state, I couldn't show up in public anyway. In this perpetual feeling of powerlessness.

That's why I only leave the house in the late evening under the cover of darkness to dispose of the trash unobserved by the neighbors.

My only reprieve from the monotony of these ensuing days is Mia, whom I constantly call. Before lectures, after lectures, basically all the time. I'm aware that she must be annoyed by my calls, but I can't help it. I constantly think about her. How she sleeps, whether she eats, whether the numbness might disappear on its own overnight. Whether she has already told her friends. And Josh. What her future might look like with this diagnosis.

Thoughts from which I can't escape. Especially on the long evenings. When night falls outside, the loneliness becomes intensely palpable. A suffocating tightness seems intent on keeping me captive until morning.

Then Tony is there to help me through at least half an hour of phone conversation. We mainly talk about trivialities, pretending to each other that nothing significant is happening. Nothing worth mentioning. Nothing that should change our lives. Or is allowed to change it.

On the eleventh day, at ten in the morning, the phone rings. It's Doctor Richards, delivering the news I had feared but still didn't want to hear. The diagnosis is clear. Multiple sclerosis, no matter how you look at it. Next Monday Mia is supposed to go to the Neurology Day Clinic.

"She'll get infusions there, and that will help," are his words.

Therefore, two days before the upcoming infusions, Mia moves back home. Tony has also returned from his business trip by now. Finally, our home is no longer empty. I am particularly delighted that Mia is back home after two long months. Because the last two months have been difficult for me. Somehow, I couldn't get used to the idea that she doesn't live in her room anymore. That I can't see her anytime. Can't knock on her door to tell her that lunch is almost ready. Can't watch her get ready for Friday evenings with her friends from her bed. Can't hug her as she passes by. Can't remove makeup together with her in the evenings and have our mother-daughter conversations. I missed all of that so much. However, I hadn't wished for her to come back home in this way. And certainly not for such a terrible reason.

"You can always go back to your study partner's place if you feel better," I try to cheer her up on Sunday evening. If she tolerates the infusions well in the next few days, it's still a possibility.

"Well, we'll see," she only responds. But I can see that she doesn't really believe it herself.

Even as we stand at the reception desk of the Neurology Day Clinic with a referral at eight in the morning the next day, Mia seems to be growing doubtful that this treatment will be as straightforward as we initially thought.

It's expected to take about four hours, a nurse explains shortly afterward. I ask her whether we are allowed to go into the large treatment room. Only the mother, she answers. That means Tony will spend the next few hours in the hospital cafeteria, drinking one coffee after another. It is not worth driving home. The way is too far. He squeezes Mia's hand before leaving, winking at her encouragingly. That's how it is between them, it comes to my mind. Without many words.

I look around the large, brightly lit patient room of the day clinic. The walls are painted a light yellow. I like that. It reminds me of the wall color on the island. Mimosa. Then I count the beds. There must be about ten beds. Some patients are already lying in the beds, connected to an IV tube. Some read, others listen to music through their headphones. And … all of them are older than Mia. That catches my attention immediately and makes me even more pensive. A nurse comes and shows Mia a bed by the window. Her patient file is already on the nightstand. Well, at least well-organized, I think, as I glance at it briefly. Next to the nightstand is a chair, so I take a seat.

In the middle of the room is a long desk with a counter, and behind it sits a young doctor at the computer. White coat, I notice immediately. She can't be a nurse. It's very quiet in the room. Mia and I exchange glances.

"Doesn't look as bad as I thought," I whisper.

"No. But they're all older than me," she replies.

So she noticed it too, I think then, but I don't let this thought show on my face.

The nurse from earlier comes and informs us that the doctor will come in shortly to examine Mia. No need to worry, she doesn't have to undress.

So Mia sits on the bed, and we wait. I repeatedly squeeze her hand and smile encouragingly.

"I'm not nervous, Mom. You're the one who's nervous," she whispers, laughing.

Shortly afterward, Mia is thoroughly examined by the young doctor for about fifteen minutes, and she asks questions that both of us find somewhat surprising. I can tell by Mia's expression.

"Tell me, how about your bladder? Any difficulties with urination?"

"No," Mia answers hesitantly.

"Good, then please sit on the chair and tilt your head downward, so that your chin touches the chest. Do you feel anything?"

"Yes, it somehow radiates into my legs."

The doctor makes notes on a form on her clipboard.

"Now, please lie down on the bed, on your back, bend both legs, arms stretched out on the bed. Lift your left lower leg into the air, so that your leg forms a ninety-degree angle."

Mia follows her instructions. Apparently, it's about how long she can hold the leg up, as now the other leg is involved. The left one was easier, I think afterward.

After the examination, a nurse prepares the infusion for Mia. She places a syringe, needles, and bandages in a tray. We take the opportunity to discuss what we both silently wondered about earlier.

"Why the question about the bladder?" Mia asks. I can see the relief on her face that she gets to talk about this.

"No idea. Nobody says anything. Only questions are asked. I wonder about that too," I reply in our conspiratorial whisper.

Anyway, nobody here talks about symptoms, the exact treatment methods, or the possible extent of the illness. Doctors and nurses remain silent, and I can't shake the impression that they don't want to provide detailed information about prognosis or anything similar.

But I will get hold of that information, I think, as I sit next to Mia's patient bed, lost in my thoughts over the next two hours. Mia has fallen asleep by now. I hold her hand and take the opportunity to quietly observe the other patients.

In the meantime, all the beds are occupied, I notice, as a nurse interrupts my thoughts. She comes to Mia's bedside repeatedly, checking if the infusion is flowing well.

"Strange, February isn't really relapse time. Much too cold. No heat," she explains, turning the valve of the infusion tube slightly to the right.

Relapse time, I wonder, furrowing my brow. So there's a specific time when you can expect a relapse. I'll Google that tonight. *Heat*, I note in my phone. It must have something to do with the heat.

I wonder if the other patients know about it. Maybe those who have been here more often and are more familiar with the disease.

Once again, I survey the room. Every time a patient gets up and goes to the toilet with the infusion stand, I discreetly observe him or her out of the corner of my eye. I want to observe their gait and look for any visible symptoms. Because many are listed on the internet.

Over the weekend, I dared to read about the disease for the first time. The disease with a thousand faces. You've heard that many times, I thought. But I didn't know there were so many different symptoms. Walking disabilities are especially common.

That's why I pay close attention to how everyone is walking. Meanwhile, I eavesdrop on the conversations in the room.

"Just 1% milk, everything has to be low-fat," a rather overweight patient is explaining to her neighbor. The neighbor doesn't seem thrilled with the conversation, at least that's my impression. He wants to be left alone, which is evident from the fact that he's holding an open book in his hand. She keeps talking and talking, and he nods repeatedly, not saying a word, just looking at her with annoyance. I have to laugh but can't. Later, I just have to tell Mia and Tony about this, I think to myself with a smile.

Four hours later, Tony stands in the doorway of the spacious patient room and makes a gesture to ask if Mia is ready. I show him five fingers, indicating 'just five more minutes.' He points to the waiting area, where he'll be waiting. Reliable as always, I think, and smile.

March 2016

In early March, you can already hear the first birds singing through the window in the morning. This makes me happy because the heralds of approaching spring mean longer days and more light. Mia recovered quickly after the infusions. Of course, these were not just infusions with vitamin solutions or any nutritional substances. They were corticosteroids, which, by their name alone, hinted that it must be a form of cortisone.

It doesn't sound good, I thought, but if it helps. The doctors must know, and after all, the other patients are getting the same thing.

Last week, there was a follow-up appointment. This time, not with Doctor Richards, as he had advised us to switch to Doctor Harper, the specialist in demyelinating diseases in their hospital. Of course, Mia and I immediately researched what the word 'demyelinating' means.

"The myelin layer that normally surrounds our nerves breaks down. This exposes the nerves," Mia then read to me from the internet.

"Yes, I know. I googled it last night," I replied contemplatively.

Doctor Harper is a luminary in his field, we were told. Only in his mid-thirties and already a lecturer, soon to be a professor. Last week we met him.

Well, a bit silent, I thought, but the main thing is that he does his job well. At least he answered all our questions. Briefly and to the point, yet informative.

"What can I eat?" Mia asked.

"Mediterranean food," was his rather laconic response.

"And is there anything we should pay special attention to? There's a lot on the internet," I wanted to know.

"No stress, no excessively heated exercise."

From that, you could draw conclusions about how things would go with Doctor Harper in the future. Nevertheless, I immediately had the feeling that we were in good hands with him. The way he sat in his small treatment room. One leg bent on the chair, jeans, a checked shirt, and glasses. He was always focused on the screen, meticulously examining all the new MRI images down to the smallest detail. I liked that right away.

"Typical hipster," was Mia's dry comment after we left the treatment room. She still found him nice, which could be deduced from her later descriptions to Tony.

"The critical Mia, who doesn't fall for the facade so easily. Well, if you find him nice, there must be something to it," Tony had responded, laughing.

And he'll know which treatment method is right for Mia, I add now in my thoughts. Even if it involves corticosteroids. The important thing is that by the third day of the infusion therapy in February, she was significantly better, and the numbness had nearly disappeared.

That's all that matters.

Now, a month after the first therapy, our daily routine has returned. Mia is visibly better. She attends her university lectures every day, Tony goes to his job at the company, and I am translating again. Also medical texts. Actually, they used to be my favorite texts, but shortly after the diagnosis, I couldn't touch them. I didn't want to see medical terminology and be constantly reminded that we now have to live with a diagnosis.

By now, it has gotten better, and I have somewhat processed the initial shock. It seems that Mia is also coping quite well with the fact that there's something accompanying her every day. Almost unnoticed yet always present. Initially, right after the diagnosis, it was different.

"I need to get used to the fact that there's something in my brain now. Inflammations. I can't see or touch them, but they're there," she once said to me in the evening, chatting in her bed, when everything was still very fresh.

The idea alone sometimes drives her crazy. But Mia is a fighter. A little Taurus, as we always say, always charging ahead like a bull. Come what may.

In kindergarten, she was the one in swimming class who, for her first swimming badge, repeatedly jumped from the pool edge into the water. Until the dive into the cold water looked just like the swim instructor wanted. Today, this perseverance serves her well, I think.

"I can imagine that you don't want to picture it exactly. But you can handle anything. Just think about how persistent you always are. Nothing and no one can bring you down," I replied with a smile, hugging her.

"Yes, I know. I'm just so afraid that I might not be able to walk someday."

"That doesn't have to happen. You shouldn't keep worrying about it," I tried to comfort her.

"Well, at least I won't be able to participate in the 'Speedy Sock'," she joked in the next moment in her typical manner, mimicking a disappointed expression.

Oh, the race 'Speedy Sock' in elementary school, I remembered and had to smile. She was so proud when I picked her up from the after-school care on that afternoon, and she could show me her certificate. It must have been in the third grade, so she was nine.

"You and your speedy sock. You're probably still proud of that, aren't you?"

"Hello, I was the fastest of all. That's quite an achievement. Especially as a girl. Not even the boys were as fast as me."

That's her, I think, recalling those moments. No hurdle is too high for her, no path too rocky.

– Chapter 2 –

May 2016

Mia's twenty-second birthday is approaching. This year, it falls on a Friday the 13th again. Just like the day she was born. Our lucky day.

"What do you actually wish for your birthday, sweetie?" I ask Mia in early May during lunch. She looks tired after the long lectures.

"Health," she jokes.

Tony and I exchange glances. Of course, it's a joke, but it stings for a moment.

"Oh, come on, what else do you wish for? Something we can actually buy. And please, don't go overboard." I wink at her. Especially now, I can't refuse her any wish. She's gotten thin since February, I think, observing her. While Tony and I continue eating, she picks at her food.

"Please, eat more, Mia. You've become quite slim. That can't be healthy," I admonish her and continue eating in silence.

I'm aware that some things in her life have thrown her off course. First, the change of her dream major, veterinary medicine, for which she had a burning passion. There was no prep course she didn't attend for the admission exam at the Faculty of Veterinary Medicine. Late in the evening, three times a week, she took the bus for an hour in the snowstorm from high school to attend the courses. Arriving home around 10 p.m., she would then go through physics and biology. Nothing was too demanding for her. She was willing to sacrifice everything for this dream. Time with friends, weekends, and her entire free time.

But she made it. The day her name was on the list of accepted candidates at the bulletin board was one of the happiest in her life. She still says that today.

Then she had to say goodbye to that dream, I think sadly. No more anatomy classes, which Mia used to rave about in the afternoons. No animal specimens in the university hallway. Overnight, everything changed. A new major, new classmates, new dreams, or rather goals that had to turn into dreams.

Four years later, I know that it still weighs on her. She placed her anatomy books on her bookshelf. In a special spot, as she says. They will always remind her that it's worth dreaming. In addition, things don't seem to be going well with Josh either. He has moved back to his hometown.

Sometimes I hear her talking to him on the phone, but afterward, she remains silent, sitting on her bed. She doesn't want to talk about it when I inquire. I understand that. That's how she has always been. She discusses things when the time is right for her. All of this is taking such a toll on her that she has hardly eaten anything lately, and that worries me.

Overall, her physical condition seems to be deteriorating. It's not just the weight loss.

Just a few days later, shortly before her birthday, she suddenly experiences a strong burning sensation in her legs in the evening. I try to alleviate the pain with cold compresses, but the burning persists. Then I give her painkillers, but that doesn't help either.

"It burns as if I dipped my legs in hot water," Mia explains to me in despair as she sits on the couch massaging her feet.

"It's probably just from your stretching exercises," Tony tries to find an explanation, but I suspect that it might be more than just muscle soreness.

Next morning, when her left leg gives way when getting out of bed, and she can't stand properly on one leg anymore, I am completely beside myself. I call the hospital, but I can't reach anyone. In the afternoon, I try again, and fortunately, Doctor Harper's receptionist answers.

"She has a strong burning sensation in both legs. She's never had this before. And since this morning, she can't stand properly on one leg," I explain anxiously to the receptionist after introducing myself.

"There's a free appointment next week," she replies kindly, but even before she finishes the sentence, I insist, "No, it has to be sooner. You don't understand. Mia can't stand anymore. We were just in hospital in February for therapy, and now it's starting again. Can't you somehow squeeze us in? Tomorrow?"

After a short pause, she responds, "Well, then come in tomorrow morning at nine, and wait until Doctor Harper has some time for you between appointments."

Okay, I think, tomorrow is fast enough. We can endure that, and then we'll see. But, I realize in the next moment, didn't Doctor Harper say that after the last corticosteroid therapy in February, Mia shouldn't undergo any further treatment for a while? How does he envision this, I wonder, feeling the first hint of panic rising in me. How long does he expect her to wait until the next treatment? Until she ends up in a wheelchair?

The same large patient room in the Neurology Day Clinic, the same nurses. This time, Doctor Harper prescribes a larger quantity of corticosteroids.

"Five days, just like in February," he instructs the head nurse.

When I later see the amount of infusion in the bag flowing through the drip into Mia's veins, I am shocked. No one in this patient room seems to require such a large quantity, and that scares me. Could it be just a precautionary measure, I wonder. Or do I need to admit to myself that the other patients are simply doing better, and the disease is not progressing as rapidly. But I keep these thoughts to myself. I won't even be able to ask Doctor Harper this question in Mia's presence without giving her the impression that I am seriously concerned about whether everything will be okay. Because that's what I repeat over and over when she casually asks me.

"Yes, of course, everything will be just fine," I reply.

What else can I say? I am her mother. The one who always has to have a bandage ready for the wound. Who should never be at a loss for an answer. No matter how difficult it is, or whether I am really sure that I know what is right. Or if I just hope so.

However, when the infusion therapy is completed after five days, my hope seems to be confirmed. This time, too, everything went as planned and without any side effects. And on the fifth and final day of treatment, Mia can even walk a little better.

It's her twenty-second birthday, and she manages to go to the bathroom on her own with the IV stand. Optimistic and joking, as always, she has completed the therapy. I admire that, I think repeatedly, as I look at her.

While she's in the bathroom, Tony helps me quickly inflate a pink balloon and attach it to her hospital bed.

The attending young doctor in the room smiles when she sees it. Typical parents, she might think. They want to bring joy to her daughter in this situation. But I don't care what others think. Whether they find it silly that I attach a balloon to the hospital bed of a young woman who is clearly beyond childhood. It's her day, and everyone can see it.

Although Mia rolls her eyes a bit when she returns from the bathroom to the patient's room, she can't hide a smile.

"Maybe I should post a photo of myself with the drip. Hashtag MS," she jokes shortly after and pretends to strike a particularly dramatic pose for the photo.

Behind these jokes and irony, there's some bitterness and fear, I see it in her gaze, and it saddens me.

While Mia is still connected to the infusion in the patient's room later, I approach Doctor Harper out of earshot. I don't want Mia to hear what's on my mind today.

"Doctor Harper, do you have a moment?" I ask him in a subdued tone, glancing repeatedly at Mia to make sure she doesn't overhear our conversation.

"Yes, sure," he responds, turning away from another patient.

"I'd like to know if there's another therapy besides these corticosteroids. I did some research, and it doesn't seem to be particularly good in the long run. Especially for the bones."

I look at him expectantly and try to interpret from his gaze what he might think about my question before he says a word. Whether he will be honest.

"There is a new medication on the market. A biologically advanced one. I would like to treat Mia with that," he explains, and in his gaze, I sense the seriousness of the following sentence. "You need to know," he continues hesitantly, "that your daughter has a highly aggressive form of multiple sclerosis, and it needs to be treated differently."

I have to take a deep breath as the meaning of his words hits me. Highly aggressive. I didn't expect that. Today, on her twenty-second birthday, this is not what I wish for my child. A future with such an illness.

"However, the health insurance must first approve the medication, and it may take some time because it involves a significant cost coverage. I've already compiled the application last week and was going to call you in the next few days. We need all the records from the past years indicating that the disease was not recognized," he further explains.

"We have plenty of those," I reply bitterly. Anger rises in me as I briefly think about all the inconclusive examinations. Couldn't any doctor put two and two together?

"It's best if you bring me all the records as soon as possible. You don't need an appointment. Tell the nurse I'm waiting for the documents."

A special medication, I think after the conversation is over and Doctor Harper leaves the patient room. Highly, it occurs to me. Highly aggressive.

Later, Mia, Tony and I are at home eating burgers. After today's final day of therapy, Mia didn't feel like having a proper birthday celebration. She's exhausted. Tony brought us fast food to celebrate. It's not healthy, but we don't care today.

The news about the new medication is a real relief for Mia, she tells me after I share my version of the conversation with Doctor Harper. Of course, I omit the words 'highly' and 'aggressive'.

"That's a great birthday gift," she jokes. "A biologically advanced medication."

In the evening, Mia and I lie together in her narrow bed and look up at the ceiling.

"Do you remember when you made me those paper butterflies and hung them in my bed canopy? We were lying like this then."

"You had just turned six and insisted on having a canopy bed in your room before starting school."

"My room? You mean our room," she replies and laughs.

"What choice did I have? Two-room apartment, single parent. Did it bother you?" I ask teasingly.

"No. I always liked it. Just the two of us, always together."

"And our children's cassette tapes before going to bed."

"Yes," she replies with a laugh, "your favorite cassette was the one with the witch and the weather frog. We listened to it over and over. And how you used to blow-dry my hair in the living room after my bath on Sundays while my show was on, and we sang the Good Night Song with the bear."

"I loved that," I smile wistfully.

She turns her head to me and looks at me.

"Mom, do you really believe in God?" she asks, almost whispering.

I hesitate because I know why she's asking, and it pierces my heart.

"Yes, I honestly believe in God, and I wouldn't pray to Him if it didn't make sense to me."

"But then why does He do this? I know that's the eternal question. Why does God allow bad things to happen? But I really want to know. Why? Did I do something wrong? Wasn't I nice enough?"

She is intelligent and knows she hasn't done anything wrong, but I've often asked myself the same question since February.

"Honestly, I don't have a proper answer to that. I can't explain it either. I mean, only three percent of the disease is said to be genetic. Three percent seems low. Environmental influences, infections. You know, what the doctors have mentioned as possible causes. But what God had in mind, I don't know."

"People always say there's a higher plan." She emphasizes the last two words, and rolls her eyes. "I just wonder what kind of plan that's supposed to be."

"You know, essentially, it doesn't help us to seek an answer to the 'why'. We have to do everything to make sure you're well. That you eat healthily. Because it surely has an impact on the inflammation. And the infusions seem to be working. Look, after five days, you're already walking much better. Now we have to make sure your walking improvement stays that way. You also shouldn't take everything to heart all the time. And everything doesn't always have to be perfect. Like at the university. Stress is not good for you."

"I know, but you just have to be able to keep up. No one asks if you're sick or feeling bad. How am I supposed to handle this if the walking issues keep coming back? And how am I supposed to live like this?"

"You'll be getting a special medication, as Doctor Harper said. One that doesn't just push the inflammation away but is biologically advanced. The health insurance just needs to approve it. It sounds promising to me."

"Yeah, that's true. After that, they say you should have peace for several years, according to the internet. That would be enough for me, for now," she responds thoughtfully.

"Who knows what new medications they'll develop in the future. Look at how far research has come for some diseases. We're doing our part to keep you healthy, and the medication takes care of the rest."

"Oh, Mom," she smiles and nestles against me, "you always find something good in everything. Classic you."

At least for this moment, I've eased her fear a bit, I think to myself.

Even if I don't have an answer to the question of why.

I hug her, inhale the scent of her hair, and wish that all of this were just a bad dream from which we could finally awaken.

June 2016

In mid-June, it's exam time at the university, but Mia won't be able to write the exams. She can no longer hold the pen with her right hand. Within just a few days, her hand has become progressively weaker. She now brushes her teeth with her left hand, but when it comes to writing, it's different. And the nerve pain in her arm is sometimes unbearable for her. This is a new symptom that we were unaware of. Only a third of MS patients experience nerve pain, Doctor Harper explained to us.

Why she has to be part of that third is a mystery to me, and Mia is not pleased either. After all, she is determined to finish the academic year. It's important to her not to fall behind, so at least these paralyzing pains must go away.

That's why, since yesterday, we have a dealer. A cannabis dealer. Because cannabis is supposed to be effective against this type of pain. "It has to be good stuff," they told us in the MS support group.

But what does good stuff look like, the three of us wonder during dinner. We have no idea, and who should we ask? There's certainly no information hotline.

"Excuse me, how should the stuff be? And how should it taste to know it's really good?" you might inquire.

It occurs to me that we need to go directly to the source. Those who really know what's good.

Sonya, the head of the MS support group is straightforward and knowledgeable. She provides "certain numbers." And the next day, the appointment with the dealer is scheduled. Since I, as a person who always follows all the rules, am not the right one for handling such substances, the family council has chosen Tony to meet with the dealer.

"Maybe you should dress accordingly," I joke as Tony prepares for the meeting.

"Yeah, like a tracksuit with a big designer logo, a hoodie, and golden sneakers," Mia suggests, laughing.

The supposed dealer turns out to be a nice middle-aged guy who also suffers from MS and just wants to help.

However, we have to determine for ourselves whether the delivered stuff is good, he says. That could take a while. Mia is supposed to take a little bit of a kind of paste every day.

Unfortunately, the time until the upcoming exams in two weeks is too short to expect a real effect. But we cling to every straw.

Furthermore, she finds herself dragging her right leg once more. Since the last infusion therapy in May, the symptoms have not completely subsided, and that makes us impatient. Impatient about the promised medication. So that the symptoms finally go away, and everything is okay again, I keep thinking.

Another corticosteroid therapy is not possible so soon after the last treatment. We know that.

That's why the only thing that matters at the moment is that Mia's exams don't suffer. There must be a solution to how to handle taking the exams in writing. Because there is always a solution, I think, and I call Mrs. Angel, the head of the PR and Media Studies program at the university. I will have to write the exam for Mia, I explain to her. There is currently no other way out.

And so, on the first day of the exams, Mia and I arrive at the university administration office at nine in the morning to find the department head, Mrs. Angel, and one of her colleagues already there.

Tony drove us, and we entered through the back entrance. Mia didn't want her fellow students to see her in this condition. Dragging one leg and accompanied by her mother.

"I looked perfectly normal during the last lectures," she reminds me "And I don't want them to stare and gossip. You know what that is like. Everyone knows what I have, and they can put two and two together."

"Well, at least you're very well-prepared," I reply, trying to divert her thoughts from the other students.

Although preparing for the exams was truly challenging, I briefly recall the past two weeks in my mind. Mia couldn't hold the books herself.

Most of the time she was lying in her bed due to severe pain. I held the books, turned the pages for her, and marked important passages with a highlighter. She is an excellent learner, and I know she must have felt somehow humiliated by losing that independence. But the brain is still functioning, she joked repeatedly, tirelessly repeating the study material for hours. She verbally created mnemonics and meticulously went through numerous manuscript pages.

In between we had to take breaks. The nerve pain was almost unbearable at times, coming in waves. Seeing her bent forward in bed in the grip of a cramp was almost too much to bear. Yet, it didn't deter her from learning.

And now the time has come to put all her efforts on paper. We arranged with the administration that Mia would dictate the answers to the exam questions to me, and I would write them down. Since everything must follow a certain procedure, Mrs. Angel and her colleague will supervise us during the exam.

Ten minutes later, Mrs. Angel and her colleague have prepared the exam materials on the large round table.

"Well, then show what you've learned," I tease her before it starts.

I'm so nervous, as if I had to prove my knowledge here, not Mia. Yet, she will dictate, and I will just write. Hopefully, I won't make any mistakes or be too slow, I nervously think as I first write Mia's personal information on the first blank sheet.

"We'll go through the exam questions first, and feel free to ask if anything is unclear," Mrs. Angel explains briefly.

"No, I have no questions," Mia declares after flipping through the exam material, and I look at her questioningly.

Then Mrs. Angel glances at the large wall clock in the university leadership's office, and the exam begins. Mia and I exchange meaningful looks. They say 'Let's do it'. She dictates, I write.

Despite all odds, Mia passed all her exams, and her well-deserved summer break can begin. It's the end of June, and we're heading to the island to our small fishing village. Tony is from there, and I spent all my childhood summer vacations in this place. In the late seventies, my parents bought a vacation home here. Since then, we spend as much time as possible in our cozy little village. With village gossip and old grandmas always knowing what you're cooking for lunch because they watch you shop at the only store.

Mia and I go to my parents' vacation home, and Tony goes home to his parents. That's how we like it. When people ask if our arrangement works, I always say, "In the summer, we keep things modern." Surprisingly, it's usually those who have been calling each other "honey" and "darling" for years and have never spent a night apart who ask. Yet, after several years, they end up going their separate ways. Unlike us. We've been handling the summer this way for sixteen years, and everyone is happy with it. During the day, Tony and I take the boat out, and in the evenings, we meet up all dressed up like two teenagers in the village at the bridge and go out together. We like it.

I take my work with me on my laptop. Especially now, I realize what a privilege it is that I no longer have a nine-to-five job, and my office can be anywhere. Overlooking the sea or the city lights. These days, they call it being a digital nomad. Before I became self-employed, this wasn't possible. Three weeks of summer vacation was the ultimate in luxury. Hardly had the suitcases been unpacked, the house cleaned, the garden restored, the vacation was almost over. After the vacation is before the vacation, that was my constant mantra.

Now it's different. And this year, in this challenging time, we particularly need the peace of village life. I yearn for everything that used to bother me about this supposed village idyll. For the familiar in this small village cosmos. Here, the world is still in order. At least on the surface.

However, that's enough for me at the moment for my idea of seclusion, far away from the clinic. And the diagnosis, I think as we arrive and I inhale the scent of pine and sea breeze.

But we carry that with us, I smile bitterly, reflecting on the brief, carefree moment when I thought we could escape it.

A few days after our arrival, my mother arrives. Since my father's death, we only spend the summer as a trio. One is missing, and each of us still feels it. In every corner of the house. In the garden, where he used to plant his tomatoes in neat rows every summer, their clusters smelling of genuine tomato fruit when picked. In the scent of the pines, reminding me of the long evening walks after ice cream in my childhood. In the song of the birds, whose names he knew for some reason and told stories about them. Memories of him are everywhere.

Much has changed since his death twelve years ago. We've been renting out the upper apartment in the house to guests from around the world for several years now. Initially, it was a bit unfamiliar. Each guest requires a different approach. And we've really had a few things to adjust to.

He's old, she's young. She looks brand new again, and he's still young and fresh. You do give a strange look when the booking only says *2 adults*, and the guests get out of the car.

Oops, where's the husband? There's the grandpa who traveled with them, you think and try to hide the initial surprise from the guest. Last year, we had an older, freshly restored doctor from Switzerland who had arrived with her much younger lover. It wouldn't have been so out of place if she hadn't behaved like a fifteen-year-old. Doors were slammed, she sat sulking on the bed when I came to check on things. She was in a fight with him, she said, and pointed her finger at her traveling companion. And she couldn't chat with other men in the bedroom because the internet connection was disturbed by the rain.

Well, that's life on an island, I thought, but said something else. "Oh, it can't be all that bad…" and "Enjoy your vacation while you're here."

Her assortment of pills on the bedside table revealed a deeper story. I didn't want to interfere, but they were sleeping right above our heads, and that's why you wish for a little harmony for your guests.

That's also why we're especially looking forward to hopefully easygoing travelers this summer, who have their emotions somewhat under control. Therefore, the vacation home needs to be spruced up. My Excel spreadsheet with all the pending tasks comes into play, and we could get started if it weren't for Mia feeling nauseous every morning since last week.

Regardless of what she ate the night before, how well she slept, or what she does during the day. She constantly has to throw up. Although walking and the weakness in her right hand have significantly decreased in the first few days on the island, the vomiting is new. I'm concerned about this unexpected nausea, which we initially can't explain.

July 2016

The constant nausea has been going on for a full four weeks now. According to Doctor Harper, some patients might experience these side effects after corticosteroid therapy, but only for a few days. I called from the island shortly after the vomiting started. This may sometimes happen. Perhaps it's due to one of the inflammation spots in the brain.

"So there's a specific spot responsible for nausea," Mia dryly commented.

By now, she's well-informed about every aspect of the disease. She knows all her MRI images and can correlate each inflammation spot in the brain with specific symptoms. I admire her for that. How fearlessly she examines everything, viewing it on the computer from a CD. I often think I couldn't do that myself. I'd probably want to close my eyes. Don't look until it's over. But it doesn't just pass by so easily, this multiple sclerosis.

"When can we expect the medication?" I asked Doctor Harper.

"That all depends on the health insurance, as I mentioned before. First, a certain procedure must be followed. The Pharmacy and Therapeutics Committee reviews all the documents and then examines whether Mia is eligible for the medication."

I knew the costs were significant. Two treatments within two years are necessary, and the total costs are about eighty thousand dollars. It's not cheap, but we're holding onto it because, according to international studies, it brings a significant improvement in symptoms and prevents the disease from progressing so far. And that's what it's all about for me. It's about finally stopping the disease's progression.

Thanks to Mia's research, we now also know what the medication is made from: a rat antibody discovered in Cambridge. She jokes that she has no problem with that, as she likes animals in every variation. The main thing is for the medication to finally arrive.

However, the days pass, and nothing happens. Every time my cell phone rings, my heartbeat skips a beat. After all, it could be the crucial call. No matter where I am, my phone is constantly within reach. Whether it's in the morning on the terrace with coffee or in the afternoon on the beach, I continuously check to see if I might have missed a call.

By the end of July, the wait becomes almost unbearable, and I call the clinic. They kindly explain to me that the Pharmacy and Therapeutics Committee of the health insurance company only meets on Thursdays, and now the vacation season is starting. "What does that mean?" I almost shout into my cell phone. Although I know the friendly lady on the other end has nothing to do with the approval process.

"But there must be a way to resolve the matter," I try to say more politely.

"I'm sorry, but there's nothing we can do about it. You just have to be patient. As soon as we get approval from the health insurance company, we'll call you and schedule a therapy appointment for Mia."

So, they want me to be patient. To be patient even though my child vomits every morning, constantly experiences pain, and cannot participate in life like any other young woman. Her friends go out to clubs in the evenings, but my daughter can't even get past putting on make-up. She puts on make-up, wants to get dressed, but then she goes back to the toilet bowl. After that, she sits on the living room couch, exhausted and drained, with smeared mascara. Still in her underwear. That's when she lies down, and Grandma and Mom try to comfort her. We know things are tough right now, but trust us, it will get better, we say.

Once the medication arrives.

My mother is visibly struggling with the whole situation. She is a tough woman, not spoiled by life. Nevertheless, she has always gone her way, never let herself be defeated by the adversities of life. She took care of my father until the very end. In his final year, he was already in a wheelchair due to a muscular disease he had suffered from for years.

It wasn't easy for her. And now, she has to go through it all again with her only grandchild, I often think when I look at her in an unobserved moment.

We don't live in the same city, and summer marks the start of our time together. It's not always easy. Three generations under one roof. Grandmother, daughter and granddaughter. Each with a personality of her own. Any potential differences are quickly resolved because we want to make living together pleasant. We avoid disputes we might have if we lived in the same city and saw each other more often. If we had more time together, we could sometimes afford to have these disputes and not talk to each other.

However, we avoid that to have a pleasant time. Although we are fundamentally different.

My mother comes from a generation that cares a lot about what the neighbors think. This bothers her even more now. Everyone in the village already knows that "the granddaughter of…" has MS. People whisper seemingly inconspicuously when my mother is in line at the cash register at the village store to do her shopping. Someone might casually ask how the family is doing. But no one wants to be the first to bring up the specific topic.

The cashier has it easier in this regard. While scanning items on the conveyor belt, she can ask.

"Anything else for you?" she asks as the opening question, looking friendly.

"No, thanks."

"When did you arrive?"

"Last week."

"Then you'll probably stay for the whole summer, right?"

"Yes, probably."

At this point, the crucial question about the well-being of the family is expected. The other villagers in line behind my mother have already perked up their ears and are eagerly waiting.

"And how are you doing?" the cashier asks, looking attentively around.

This is the moment when people in line move a little closer to not miss anything. Even if it means Mrs. Davis presses her shopping basket into Mrs. Miller's aching back. After all, everyone wants to catch every detail to join the conversation later or be the first to share the latest gossip on the bench outside the post office.

"Good," my mother responds while paying.

Pay, pack, and get out, offering no material for village gossip in the days to come. Smile politely and leave.

My mother gets upset about it. She lives in the big city. She always says you can have peace and quiet there, away from all of this. Unfortunately, you can't escape the village customs here. You quickly get caught up in the maelstrom of village life, whether you want to or not. Sometimes you have to provide information just to quiet the chatty village women. And that skill has to be learned. Give a short answer, a polite smile, and keep going.

Of course, right after my mother leaves the store, someone says, "Oh, she didn't look too good."

"Haven't you heard about her granddaughter?"

"No, what happened?" Heads lean in, whispering to share information cautiously, savoring the details for later. Otherwise, the magic of later retelling fades too quickly.

"Well, she's dealing with that illness that affects her mobility. She's probably using a wheelchair by now."

"That's terrible. Have you seen her?"

"No, not yet, but I might stop by for coffee in the next few days."

"Sure, do that. I'm too busy for it, but send my best wishes."

Then they appear concerned because keeping up the façade of charitable grace is always a priority. Even among themselves, they won't openly admit that they're stopping by for coffee out of curiosity. That's not appropriate. After all, they believe in God, and He sees everything. They want to be able to show their faces in church on Sunday, even if their church visit is more about exchanging village stories and seeing who else is there.

– Chapter 3 –

August 2016

In the first week of August, the long-awaited call from the clinic finally comes. The health insurance has approved the medication. But by now, Mia can no longer walk independently.

A week ago, it was just a normal day at the beach. Mia was feeling fine and didn't have any nausea that day. I think the sun must have caused it. Strong sunlight triggers relapses, they say. Mia just felt like going to the beach, like in the normal course of life. We dressed in beach attire and carried our chic fabric bags. First, the beach, then coffee on the sunny terrace of the nearby hotel overlooking the sea.

She drinks mineral water, and I have a cappuccino with vanilla flavor. As always, we enjoy this ritual, observing the tourists around us. Older female tourists lie by the large outdoor pool, trying to read books, while children jump from the pool's edge, joyfully calling out, "Look, Mommy!" The older women look up occasionally, slightly annoyed at the interruption.

At a table next to us, a couple sits in large rattan chairs. She tries to see what he is constantly typing on his phone, irritably asking if he's texting someone. He excuses himself, claiming it's just a message from the office he needs to respond to. Mia and I exchange knowing smiles.

At another nearby table, two couples who apparently arrived from England are sitting together. They all wear wedding rings and you can see their years of familiarity. He orders for her, and she plucks a pine needle from his hair.

The other couple briefly discusses who showers first before dinner. Then they engage in conversation, sharing old vacation stories and debating who had the better last vacation and who got especially tan this time.

When one couple says goodbye to take a nap before dinner, gossip starts. The couple who stayed in the café doesn't find Karen and Peter as amusing as they pretended. And actually, they are quite different, she says. Especially regarding the political views discussed during last night's dinner at the hotel. But for the vacation, they get along well enough.

As always, Mia and I enjoy these snapshots while sitting comfortably in the café.

Yet, two days later, Mia can no longer get out of bed without assistance. She says she has no feeling in her legs.

Monday, August 8, 2016. After months of waiting, the long-awaited antibody therapy begins at the Neurology Day Clinic.

We traveled by car from the island, and it was by no means easy. After all, it's midsummer, and there are still numerous tourists around. There's a lot of pushing and shoving. Their only concern seems to be making their way forward and finding a suitable seat in the deck salon of the car ferry. The heat is getting to everyone, and nervousness sets in as soon as a suitcase, a child, or, in our case, we are in their way. Overall, everything is now very challenging for us.

Tony parked the car down in the ferry at the assigned spot. Now, two options are available to get to the deck in the salon. Using the more distant elevator or the escalator a few meters away from the car. We opt for the escalator.

Tony and I support Mia as she walks. Unfortunately, the escalator isn't working when we finally get to it. It never bothered us on previous trips with this ferry. Now, it almost makes me lose my temper. The tourist queue behind us is pressing, with everyone looking frustrated, waving, and shouting for us to keep moving.

"How?" I shout into the crowd. "The escalator isn't working, and my daughter can't just walk up the damn stairs."

Tony tries to calm me down. We could try the elevator, he suggests.

I would prefer to stand still in protest at the escalator. To show the crowd that this is no walk in the park. That they should all put themselves in our situation. But it's useless. We have to try the elevator. Which means we have to walk all the way back.

Mia is sweating, she is visibly exhausted. Tony offers to carry her, but she doesn't want that. What if someone sees her? Someone who knows her. She'd be embarrassed by that. So we walk to the elevator, then sit for two hours in the salon, hoping it will all be over soon.

Just get there, I think the whole time, and watch through the window as we move further away from the island toward the mainland. Just get there. The medication is there. That's all that matters. Nothing else is important. No ignorant tourists, no weird looks.

Only that she finally gets the medication. Then everything will be okay again.

Actually, Mia was supposed to receive the medication through infusions in the Neurology Day Clinic for five consecutive days. In the afternoons, she could then go home. Instead, the doctors decide that she must be admitted to the hospital. Due to her condition, they say.

In the Neurology Unit, in the small patient room number 9, a young woman is already lying in bed when Mia is wheeled into the room in a wheelchair. Only two beds, I think relieved. Although her roommate is young, she doesn't look good, I think as I look closer. But maybe they'll talk later, then time will pass more quickly.

"Also MS," a nurse whispers to me at the door, nodding toward the young woman.

Her tone makes it sound like this young woman has the plague. Like it's highly contagious. Something to be ashamed of. As if such patients should be isolated together.

But she probably doesn't mean it that way, I think a moment later. I've just become sensitive and pay attention to every detail, every incorrectly emphasized word, every not nice enough-seeming look.

About an hour later, Mia is prepared in the hospital bed. Doctor Harper briefly enters the room and asks how Mia is doing.

"Well, I could be better," she replies.

He doesn't miss the humor in her voice, and he just nods with a smile as he signs something on a sheet. Probably his approval that the therapy can start, I think. Mia had already signed earlier, agreeing to everything that happens here. With all possible risks, all side effects.

However, not much was said about the side effects. Problems with the thyroid, the next five years, blood tests must be monitored every month. Nothing more was disclosed. On the internet, it sounded different to us. Especially Mia, who has read a lot. Hair loss and fever were the least of it. Some studies mentioned anaphylactic shock and even death.

"Well, that doesn't sound too great. I'd say I'd prefer having MS to being dead," Mia casually remarked.

She takes everything with humor, I think now. On the other hand, I feel nauseous just thinking about what could happen.

At the foot of her bed, I notice a small table with an open plastic bowl. Various medications and other supplies are inside. Probably the emergency kit if an unwanted side effect happens, it occurs to me. That scares me, but I don't show anything in front of Mia.

A nurse places the IV access a few minutes later while I sit at the foot of Mia's bed and observe everything calmly. Meanwhile, Tony has to wait outside.

It's not visiting hours now, the head nurse just explained to me, but I can stay in the patient's room until the IV is set up.

Then I have to leave. Tomorrow from four to five. That's the visiting time we should please adhere to.

Okay, understood, I think irritated. I understand that it's not visiting hours now, but this is an exceptional case. After all, my daughter is getting THE medication. We've been waiting for months, and now I'm supposed to just leave. I can't even watch as it flows into her body through the infusion and imagine how it takes effect. How it makes her healthy. A medication that looks like a simple liquid in small bottles. So inconspicuous, I think. It could also be ordinary pain drops from the drugstore.

But what did I expect, I ask myself then. A large package wrapped in gold paper? Just because it's so important to us? Because we attribute a miraculous effect to the medication and hope that the mentioned prognosis of about ten years without new relapses will last much longer. But no matter what we imagine or hope for, according to international studies, it's supposed to work.

And we firmly believe in it.

In the next few days, Tony and I visit Mia every afternoon. More or less during visiting hours. Most of the time, however, we're already standing at the entrance to Neurology Unit VI half an hour before. Through the glass door, I impatiently look for a nurse who could open the door for us ahead of time.

When we enter room number 9 shortly after, Mia has usually been on the drip for several hours. During our first visit, I was a bit surprised by the aluminum foil around the infusion tube. Meanwhile, I know it serves to protect the medication because it's light-sensitive. You never stop learning.

Today, Tony and I brought Mia lunch from home and a few bottles of water. Mia explained on the first day in the hospital that the food isn't great. That's why she can't wait for us to visit. Especially when you have to wait to be fed because the right hand is no longer working.

"Infusion in the left arm, the right one refuses to work," she jokes. "With Eva, it's the exact opposite. The whole left side doesn't want to cooperate. Leg and arm, just like me." She gestures toward the young woman in the room. "Two healthy halves combined, and we'd be whole again."

Typical Mia, I think, smiling at her grotesque remarks.

"Look, Tony, I have a private toilet now." She points to a chair with an opening in the seat next to her bed.

"Oh, how convenient. You won't have to go far. That would be something for home when watching football," he responds in the same manner.

"Eva only gets corts. They supposedly still don't know what she has. Typical doctors—it's pretty obvious," Mia explains, while Eva nods in agreement.

"Didn't they perform a lumbar puncture on you?" I inquire.

"No, not yet," Eva answers quietly.

"Well, they'll probably do it. You're in good hands here." I don't want to unsettle the young woman with my questions. She looks a bit frightened, so I change the subject.

"And how long have you been here?" I ask, putting on my reassuring motherly smile.

"Two weeks. I get corts every day."

They even have a nickname for corticosteroids here, I think, furrowing my brow. Probably a common practice among the nurses to downplay the medicine so it doesn't sound so bad. Especially for the younger patients.

When Eva has fallen asleep a bit later, I finally have the chance to ask Mia what has been on my mind since the morning.

"Was Doctor Harper at the morning rounds? And what did he say? Is everything going normally with the medication?"

"Yeah, he was here briefly. Didn't say much. If something were wrong, I'd know."

Later, I think I'll ask the head nurse more details, but for now, I say nothing.

"How are you feeling? Your face is all red, like with corticosteroids."

"The infusion has been running for a few hours. I feel tired. And this whole feeding situation is really getting on my nerves. I'd rather eat with my own hands. I got my lunch cold today because I had to wait until the nurses finished with the unit."

"And what is Eva like?" I ask softly, trying to change the subject.

"Nice. She's a year younger than me. Probably she also has MS. No one says it, but the symptoms speak for themselves. Her boyfriend visits her every day."

I know that this last piece of information is particularly tough for Mia, as her boyfriend Josh now lives in another city. They talk on the cell phone occasionally, but not frequently, and that's particularly challenging for her right now.

On the fourth day of the therapy, Mia is visibly better. She practiced walking with Eva in the hallway today. With Mark, the male nurse.

"I doubt it's already the medication," I tell Tony later in the car on the way home. "It's probably more from the corticosteroids she gets before each infusion."

"The crucial thing is that she's making progress. It's important for her to see improvement," he replies.

And he's right. We know that the effects of the medication may take one or two months. What's important to us now is that Mia leaves the clinic on her own two feet and can go back to university in October. Because that's what she keeps talking about. She worries about what might happen if she can't walk by then. or can't write again, or who knows what else might occur by fall. After all, it's only two months away, and a lot can happen in that time.

October 2016

The university has started again. Mia is doing remarkably well. Apparently, the medication has kicked in, and we couldn't be happier.

"Finally back to the routine," she says happily. "I love the fall, the early mornings when it's still dark outside. I've really had enough of summer, it's time for some rain and I can get my fall clothes out of the wardrobe."

She particularly liked fall as a child, I remember.

Back then, I was a single parent and working. In the early mornings, we would leave our apartment, which was in the middle of a park, while it was still dark outside. Mia in her small, colorful rain boots and her pink raincoat. She wanted to walk through every colorful pile of leaves on the way to the kindergarten, and I let her.

Only children have that special, contagious joy, I always thought. Even when I was in a hurry and constantly under time pressure to catch my subway and make it to the office on time. Because those brief moments were too precious for me to let them slip away. After all, these were the moments that allowed us to start the day in our own magic.

During the winter months, we were always the first in our neighborhood to leave the house in the morning. Only our footprints on the fresh blanket of snow would be seen by the next neighbor when he stepped out of the house. And those of the little birds. Mia always enjoyed that particularly. She loved leaving her own boot prints next to the tracks of the little birds.

I nostalgically think back to that time in this first autumn with MS. Back then, I was carefree. Today, however, after nine months with the diagnosis and Mia's constant setbacks, that lightheartedness seems lost.

Even as we sit in Doctor Harper's treatment room at the Neurology Day Clinic in mid-October, I feel this constant heaviness within me. A fear that keeps me on constant guard, always anticipating the next piece of bad news.

But Doctor Harper smiles as he reviews the latest MRI scans, and Mia reports that she's doing very well.

"After the therapy, I had a rash for just one day. You know I went to the emergency room because of it. I had red, big welts. But they were gone after two days. And I also have hair loss," she explains to him.

"That can happen," he murmurs, looking at the results again.

And shortly after, he bids us farewell with a smile at the door.

"That all sounds very encouraging, Mia. See you in six months. If anything comes up before, you can come earlier."

Six months of peace and no clinic visits—I think happily as we walk to the car, where Tony is already waiting. Finally, a chance to catch our breath.

December 2016

On the first weekend of Advent, it's snowing heavily outside. Mia and I are sitting in the kitchen, sipping on hot ginger tea. I've been trying to convince her for days that it's good for inflammation.

"Mia," I ask cautiously, "is there something wrong with your right leg? You seem to be walking differently than usual." I blow into the hot cup and watch her reaction out of the corner of my eye.

"I don't know. Since yesterday, I've been having trouble climbing the stairs at the university. Maybe it's just from constantly running up and down. You know how it goes—lecture, break, lecture. In between, I also have to grab a bite to eat."

She doesn't seem concerned, I think as I look at her. Nevertheless, I'll keep an eye on it.

"Okay, if anything changes, just let me know."

But just a few days later, I notice that Mia is dragging her right leg a bit. Again, I think sadly. We've recovered a bit from the whole thing, and it's starting again. Right before Christmas. Hopefully, it will go away on its own. Or should I call Doctor Harper and ask for an appointment? I contemplate back and forth.

In the end, I do schedule an appointment with Doctor Harper and can hardly believe what he uncovers. It's a psychologically induced paralysis, he explains after thoroughly examining Mia two days later. It has nothing to do with a new lesion.

"My suggestion would be for you to talk to a psychiatrist. We can arrange an appointment with a very nice colleague of mine if you want. She also works here at the clinic."

She's not exactly thrilled, I think, as Mia looks at me with our familiar gaze.

"Great, now it's even psychological. Here we go again," she later complains at home, quite displeased with this fact.

"Who knows how long this will take. They can't just get rid of it with corticosteroids. I have to do something about this, and I have no idea what that's supposed to be. I'm relaxed, what else am I supposed to do?" she asks, and her desperate expression makes me sad.

Of course, she's upset, I think then. Doctor Harper believes it might last longer. The mental blockage needs to be resolved. Through conversations where she finally unburdens her sorrow. As if we don't constantly talk about 'our sorrow' at home. We wake up with our sorrow and go to sleep with it. What does a doctor really know, I wonder for the umpteenth time. Besides, Mia has had enough of talking about 'the illness and everything else,' as she puts it. A blockage is the last thing she needs right now.

"A Blockage? No way it's just a blockage. I got through the exams, can finally walk normally again, and now this," she vents her frustration.

You never get a break from this illness, I think, shaking my head. But we have no other choice. She'll have to go for talk therapy if she wants to get back on track.

And then there's Christmas.

The matter of Christmas has to be tackled now, I've been thinking for a week. Despite the situation with Mia. All the windows in the neighborhood are already brightly lit. Everyone is trying to outdo each other with their Christmas decorations. But my usual pre-Christmas euphoria seems to have disappeared this year. I'd rather leave Christmas in the box down in our basement. The decorating, all the decor, it all seems too exhausting to me. I simply can't muster any excitement for the upcoming Christmas holiday.

On the other hand, I don't want to spoil us—especially Mia—this Christmas. It should be as usual for her. Peaceful and cozy. With the scent of cookies and the sounds of old Christmas classics.

As far as that's possible this year, I think, and chuckle at the amount of kitsch I seem to associate with Christmas.

In the end, on the third Sunday of Advent, I decide to delve into my cookie recipes. My annual cookie baking season should have started last weekend. So, it's time for me to at least begin selecting the appropriate recipes. Following that, I compile a list of ingredients for all the cookie recipes.

But, with the first vanilla cookie recipe, I hit a snag after the third ingredient. Sugar is okay; I can substitute that. However, what do I do with the eggs? I can't use them anymore. No sugar, no white flour, no vanilla sugar, and no egg yolk. Because that's also problematic, I've read. It contains a lot of Vitamin D, which is good, but too many fatty acids, which, in turn, are not good for Mia. But some binder has to go into these cookies.

So, I turn to Google. I read about using banana as a binder. That means all the cookies will taste like banana this Christmas. Banana-vanilla cookies, banana black and white cookies, banana coconut clusters, banana rum balls. That's not how I envisioned it. But I don't know how to handle it quickly in any other way.

On top of that, Tony's parents have announced their visit for Christmas Day, as they do every year. It's nice, but how will this work with the Christmas dinner now, I wonder. I browse the internet for suitable festive recipes. Unfortunately, under 'Anti-inflammatory diet' and 'Diet for MS', I can't find a completely normal recipe. I need Grandma's kitchen, just MS-friendly.

Well, I think, then I'll have to sit down for an afternoon and rewrite my recipes. Anti-inflammatory without being appetite-inhibiting, so to speak. Especially at Christmas, when you have to repeatedly showcase your cooking skills to your mother-in-law. I should be indifferent about it this year, but the perfectionist in me doesn't allow any deviation from the expected norm. It has to taste perfect.

My red cabbage is now transformed into Stevia red cabbage with frozen berries. Forget about frying onions in butter and adding two heaping tablespoons of sugar. That's now a thing of the past. Just like our previous life is a thing of the past.

Our life at Christmas without a diagnosis.

One day before New Year's Eve, Mia ends the long-distance relationship with Josh. The relationship had lasted a whole two years.

"I just called him and told him I don't want this anymore," she says to me afterward.

We're sitting on her bed in the evening. She's crying bitterly. Of course, she's crying, I think to myself. She always gave everything for this relationship. Her love, her time, her entire energy, sacrificed to make it work. To make her long-distance relationship last. And above all, to make him love her. Especially despite the illness. Now she's devastated, at the end of her strength. Because love should have helped her. It should have provided comfort from afar.

"He just didn't get it. Nothing. That the illness doesn't just go away. That I'm still the same despite it. That he can't just move away because I need him," she tries to explain desperately.

I hug her, wipe the tears from her face, but she can hardly calm down. Then she looks at me.

"Why can't this just pass, Mom? I want my old life back."

In her eyes, I see the deep pain over what she has to endure. Over the lost love that was supposed to be eternal. Over the suffering that her life with Multiple Sclerosis brings. Over the past year. And the fear of the future. An uncertain future, despite the medication.

– Chapter 4 –

January 2017

"Mom, next week, I have that job interview at the marketing agency. Do you think I should mention that I have MS, or should I just keep quiet?" Mia shouts from the apartment hallway as she puts on her boots on a cold winter morning.

It's a Monday, sometime in late January. She's on her way to the university and needs to hurry to catch her bus at five past seven.

"Good question," I reply, joining her in the hallway. "I need some time to think about it. Let's talk about it tonight."

"Okay. You know I really want this job. For my career. Anyway, see you later. Love you, Mom." She gives me a kiss on the cheek.

"Love you too, sweetie. Have fun at university," I reply, giving her a quick hug.

As I close the door behind her, I linger in the hallway, closing my eyes and smiling as I breathe in the scent of her perfume. It carries the essence of her freedom, her young life, and the happiness in her eyes as she leaves the house. And that makes me happy.

I now have every reason to be. Because she's doing well again. The leg paralysis lasted only two weeks. After the Christmas break, Mia had one session with the psychiatrist and didn't want to go back.

The psychiatrist asked if something was bothering her and encouraged her to talk about it. Mia found her competent and nice, but yet insisted it made no sense. After all, she could discuss her problems at home. She considered it a waste of time.

In retrospect, I don't mention what I think was the reason for this psychological blockade: that the situation with her ex-boyfriend weighed on her more than she wanted to admit. The fact that he wasn't there for her, and she constantly waited for his call and encouragement, must have been particularly tough for her.

This was especially true during her time in the hospital, where she had Eva and her devoted boyfriend constantly in view.

Now, after breaking free from that relationship, she's doing better. She seems more relaxed and is making plans for the future.

Next Monday, she wants to start exercising again. Cross-training and yoga. You can see her enthusiasm and zest for life.

"Look, I'm quite flexible," she explained last night in her room while attempting to pull one leg behind her head.

"Well, you won't get it behind your head," I laughed, "but it'll be enough for the beginner classes. But tell me, won't this cross-training be too strenuous for you? You've just recovered," I asked, trying not to let my concern show.

"I'll just give it a try, and if it's too much, I can always do something else. You know I can't stand lame workouts. I'll do cross on two days and yoga on Saturdays to relax," she explained.

"Always giving it her all. Typical Mia. But okay, go ahead and check it out. Just if it's too strenuous, you really have to stop."

I say this because I know her all too well. I know how it goes with her. She's stubborn, which often keeps her from admitting things to herself. Especially when it's about accepting that something might not work out or a goal might be out of reach.

Now, when it's not just about any desire but her health, we need to recognize the limit in time. Her body should not overheat or be overburdened; otherwise, it could lead to another relapse.

I hope she takes things slowly. On the other hand, I understand her. She has just recovered from everything and wants to enjoy life to the fullest.

She wants to move forward, look ahead. A part-time job alongside university is a welcome change—and a potential entry into the professional world.

And with exercise, she wants to work on her fitness again, she says. The toned bikini body must come back after the muscles suffered from constant sitting and lying down.

Certainly, she cares a lot about her appearance, I know that. Especially because she wants to keep up with her hashtag generation. Constantly, great photos are posted on the internet, likes are counted, and presented to each other.

Not only is your own success measured by it, but also the supposed happiness associated with it. The more amazing the photos, the happier your own life seems.

In the breaks between lectures, students stand together in the university halls, pointing at filtered photos, showcasing what they have to offer in life. Especially the young women. You are beautiful, you have the perfect boyfriend, you travel around the world during semester breaks, and constantly wear new outfits. Not a weekend goes by without being in a trendy club or another representative place.

Everything must be constantly captured in mobile photos. "Pics or it didn't happen" is the motto. But how do you follow this constant pressure to conform when life isn't so perfect? I often ask myself that lately when Mia asks for my opinion on a photo.

She also likes to post a nice photo of herself and then enjoys the approval of her followers.

People leave comments like 'gorgeous' or 'awesome' under her photos. But she says she doesn't measure herself by that; after all, she has other things to offer in life. She's studying for a reason and not just turning to the job of an "influencer" like many in her circle of friends.

However, I see that she does care to some extent about what others think of her and her lifestyle.

"Every now and then, I can post something, especially when something beautiful happens in my life," she says in those moments. "No one wants to see the unpleasant sides," she adds jokingly. And then I wonder how all this hashtag behavior could affect her in the future if the disease possibly reveals its less attractive side.

I also doubt that she truly doesn't care about it all. It's almost become a trend to share your life with the public through photos on the internet. And it has to be done regularly to keep up. Regardless of your current state of mind.

Around two o'clock, Tony and I grab lunch while Mia's still at the university.

"What do you think about whether Mia should mention that she has MS during the job interview next week or not?" I ask.

"Hmm," he responds, furrowing his brow as he continues to eat. "That's not so easy to answer. On one hand, it might make it harder for her to get the job because they'll only think about the potential absences. On the other hand, the employer will find out anyway. At least with the first sick leave."

"Well, you're right," I say, pondering. "The employer can also identify it from the diagnosis code. That means we'll have to think about how she can best handle it during the interview."

When Mia comes home late in the evening, I bring up her question from this morning. She's exhausted from the long lectures but brimming with anticipation for the upcoming job interview.

"As for your interview at the marketing agency, we need to come up with a plan on how to incorporate MS into the conversation. I mean, I wouldn't mention it right at the beginning of the interview, but you do need to bring it up," I suggest.

"Well, then I can probably forget about the job. Employers don't want someone who's sick and might be absent," she replies, taking off make-up at her make-up table. I sit on her bed watching her. Finally, she's back here with me, briefly crosses my mind.

"I would say you need to convince them first with your knowledge and then bring it up. Maybe, the best time would be when you're asked why you switched from veterinary medicine to PR and Media Studies. That's when you can bring up the topic of MS."

"The question is, what exactly should I say then?" she responds, turning to me briefly. "By the way, I have MS. But fortunately, there's a fantastic medication I've been taking, and I'm doing really well now," she says.

"Something like that. You're eloquent. Come up with something brief so the employer doesn't dwell on the topic for too long," I suggest, smiling encouragingly.

"Then, I'll just say I had to change my major because I have MS. Now, I'm doing great, and I'm highly motivated."

"Well, that sounds good. And then you can steer the conversation in a different direction."

"But once I've said it," she says, "the question is whether they still want me. Who knows what such job interviews will look like for me in the future, when it's no longer about a student job. Fortunately, this job is only for three months, so they might not worry too much about whether I might feel worse in the future," she adds.

"You're confident. You have to radiate that. Just focus on your strengths. And you know what… even if this employer rejects you, the next employer might see things differently."

Deep down, I hope that there will be an employer who at least considers their so-called 'employment quota' and overlooks the fact that Mia has MS. Even though this thought saddens me. Who would have thought that it would come to this, that I have to rely on an employer's pity in Mia's job search? I, too, should focus on her strengths and follow her example—staying positive.

That's how Mia got her first student job a week later. The interview actually went roughly as we had planned.

At some point, the question arose as to why she had changed her majors. That was exactly the sticking point in her still short CV that her potential employer could ask about. Everything else, however, is exemplary. Excellent grades, outstanding high school GPA, proficiency in multiple languages. There's nothing to criticize in those areas.

Only this tiny yet conspicuous irregularity, this twist, cannot be overlooked. Why would a veterinary medicine student switch to PR and Media Studies, you might ask yourself as an employer. After all, it's known that meeting the requirements for a spot at the University of Veterinary Medicine is no easy feat. And then, she simply stops and chooses something else?

The same question probably crosses an employer's mind, and I'm relieved that Mia was prepared for it, smoothly navigating through her response.

I don't want to imagine how much it would have exposed her if she suddenly had to explain herself. If she didn't know whether to lie and say she didn't enjoy veterinary medicine. Or if the moment had come to reveal herself.

To expose her innermost self and say: "I have MS."

And then to see the question marks over the heads of the interviewers. Realizing the conversation might be over because a decision has already been made. Even before before the entire job interview process has been completed.

However, she was spared from all of that, and I'm relieved that now her plans for the future can move forward. A new student job is a good start.

But… what if she gets worse again? I often think these days that from one day to the next, she might not be able to walk anymore. With that feeling, I now bid her goodbye every morning at the apartment door. And I hope that no text or call reaches me, where she anxiously tells me that something is numb again and everything is starting over.

March 2017

Mia has been working at the marketing agency for a month now, attending classes at the university, and hitting the gym four times a week in the evenings. In between, she manages to meet up with her friends when time allows. You can tell how fulfilled she is.

She leaves the house happily in the morning and returns home after cross-training in the evening—exhausted but still full of energy.

Of course, I worry if it's all too much at once. But I keep my concerns to myself. And at dinner in the evening, Tony and I listen to what she has to tell us about her day.

However, Mia only tells me when we're alone and getting ready for bed in the bathroom that her coworker Ben, who's her age, wants to invite her for coffee. She explains with a smile that it's not something for Tony's ears.

"Well, here's the question again: Do I tell him or not? And if I do, should I bring it up during our first coffee or wait? I mean, he looks good and seems to like me, but will that change if he knows?" she ponders aloud. Sitting on the bathroom floor in front of the mirrored cabinet, she removes the eyeshadow from her eyes with a cotton pad.

"Actually, you don't owe anyone your personal details right off the bat. That's nobody's business," I reply, perching on the edge of the bathtub. "I mean, it sounds as if you have some terrible flaw you need to disclose immediately. Like a contagious infection."

"Yeah, I know. As long as the illness isn't visible, it's okay. I'm not limping or anything. But it's still there, and imagine if I start a serious relationship with him, and he doesn't know. That's a breach of trust."

"On one hand, you're right. But I still wouldn't say anything during the first coffee. If you like him and you start seeing each other more often, then you can mention MS and see how he reacts," I suggest. "I mean, guys have been lining up for you, so you shouldn't worry."

"Maybe that was the case before. Now, I'll be lucky if anyone takes me with MS," she replies, and it breaks my heart to hear her say something like that about herself.

"If someone has an issue with it, then he's not worth your time. Then he's just not the right one for you. And you've got a way to filter out who's right for you and who's not by telling him about MS. Look at it this way…" I try to steer the conversation in a different direction. In my mind, I add, They say 'for better or for worse' for a reason.

I hope there's someone out there for her. Maybe grabbing coffee with this Ben is a good way to find out.

A few days later, Mia tells me somewhat hesitantly about her first coffee with Ben. It's around eleven at night, and we're in her room. She just got home and is changing.

They went to a café across the street after work in the late afternoon, she says.

She liked the atmosphere of the café ›Bonheur‹. Then she describes the mood, the dim lighting, the plush chairs. It was all very romantic.

He kept looking at her, which flattered her. He complimented her. Not only was she very pretty, he said, but also so ambitious, and he liked that. The other young women he knew were different. It was all about their looks and the parties they attended, he said.

But she wasn't just attractive, she was also intelligent. He saw that at work, he said. How she talks to customers, always takes notes, and learns faster than the others.

Well, he seems to have recognized her true qualities in a short time, I think as she tells me this.

She didn't tell him about her illness at first, she says. First she wants to see how things develop.

Then she shows me his profile picture on social media. You can tell at first glance that he likes sports. He's sitting in a sports stand and smiling. In the picture he seems likable to me.

Anyway, she feels like something could come out of it, she continues. He asked her when she was free again. For another coffee. Maybe they could go to a different café next time. One in the city where they could take a walk afterward.

May 2017

In early May, Doctor Harper wants to see what's been happening in Mia's brain since she started the medication last August. The second cycle is coming up this August, then that's it. At least that's what they're saying. Two cycles and she'll have peace for several years. No relapses, no major symptoms.

The regular life of a nearly twenty-three-year-old, I think eagerly as Mia and I sit in Doctor Harper's office a week after the new MRI scan.

"Well, there are some new lesions visible, but that was to be expected," he explains to us, focused on the MRI images on the computer screen.

For my part, I didn't expect that, I think, feeling my heart rate increase. There was never any talk of new lesions. On the contrary, they were supposed to disappear.

"When can we expect to be no more new inflammations then?" I ask, a bit louder than intended.

"After Mia receives the second cycle in August. Only then is the treatment with the medication completed," he answers, scrolling to the next image on his screen.

"I didn't notice anything from the lesions," Mia interjects. "Were they in places where it wouldn't be noticeable?" she asks Doctor Harper.

"Probably. Sometimes the inflammation spots are very tiny and in areas where the symptoms are almost imperceptible. As I said, we'll see the final results a month or two after the second dose of medication. You've been doing okay so far, right?" He looks at her.

"Yes," she replies, beaming. "I'm going to university, I've got a student job. Can't complain."

And there is a new boyfriend, I add in my mind.

"Well then, we'll see you in August," he smiles, and we leave the Neurology Clinic.

This year, Tony and I are heading to the island shortly after Mia's birthday in mid-May without her, as the first bookings for the vacation rental are coming in. Mia is staying in the city and will join us once she passes her exams and finishes her student job.

She seems visibly excited to finally have some time to herself. According to her, being alone in the apartment without parents is particularly enjoyable, as it gives her a sense of freedom.

I can already picture her picking out scented candles at the drugstore and arranging her purchases all over the apartment. She loves that. Whenever she has her own place, everything will smell like vanilla and such, she always says.

On the other hand, those scents bother me, and there's been a reason for it for the past week.

I'm pregnant. At almost forty-four years old. "You've really pulled it off," my OB-GYN almost proudly commented during the first ultrasound two days ago.

There's nothing to see yet except for a yolk sac, but it's still too early in the pregnancy for a visible embryo.

We're overjoyed about the baby. Tony, because it's his first biological child, and Mia, because she's been wishing for a sibling for a long time. I already have names picked out for a boy or a girl in my head, but I'll keep them to myself for now.

However, there's a catch that will stay with me until the end of the pregnancy. Two years ago, I was pregnant—until I started bleeding in the ninth week.

"That's just the age catching up with you, no need to wonder," my then OB-GYN explained to me unsympathetically as he performed the dilation and curettage under local anesthesia.

How considerate, I thought back then, as I lay there with tears streaming down my cheeks. "So I'm old, but I can still get pregnant," I thought.

And now it's happened again. In a time when I see this pregnancy as a real reward for all the suffering and worries that the MS diagnosis has brought us.

This time, we won't tell anyone. Only the three of us and my mother know about it. And the family council has decided to keep it that way until the twelfth week of pregnancy is over.

With this pregnancy, our euphoria won't drive us to shout it to the world, to proudly tell the whole village.

No, we'll remain silent and blissful as the baby happily grows in my belly. And I can't wait to hear the little heartbeat for the first time.

– Chapter 5 –

Saturday in June 2017

With our vacation home spruced up in the first week of June and the garden freshly dug and replanted, the arrival of our first guests this season is imminent. It's Saturday. Check-in day.

This year, my mother and I decided to get ourselves a cleaning lady. After all, I'm supposed to be taking it easy now. But I couldn't stand it for long. Cleaning is something I prefer to do myself.

People born under the zodiac sign of Virgo, like me, are meticulous, and I can't resist that urge. Everything has to be spotless.

That's why I secretly clean up after our cleaning lady leaves. While my mother calmly plants the garden with flowers carefully chosen by me from the gardener's, which were just delivered. Purple, pink, yellow, white. Red and orange flowers are out of the question. Everything should come as close as possible to my idea of an English garden.

Just like our neighbors Jane and George, who have such a garden in England. They live near London on a country estate with vast lands. Jane likes to show me photos of her garden. I can't get enough of the abundance of her roses and wildflowers.

That's exactly how I want my garden to look. At least in theory.

Shortly after five o'clock in the afternoon, Sergej and Tatjana arrive with their baby. He's twenty-three years older than her, married to her in his second marriage. They booked forty-seven nights. Tatjana's parents will come in the third week of their vacation with Sergej's four-year-old daughter from his first marriage. Eventually, a friend of Sergej's might come by too. At least that's what Sergej has planned.

Well, I think, if they're nice, forty-seven nights is great. But what if they aren't? Then it could feel like a very long time.

And my fear is confirmed just a few minutes after the guests arrive. Sergej makes his status as a guest unmistakably clear: he pays, so I should toe the line. Unfortunately, he's barking up the wrong tree, I think, as I warmly show the couple around the spacious vacation rental.

The tour starts as usual in the hallway. Then I show them the bedrooms. One with a garden view, the other overlooking the sea and with access to the terrace.

Tatjana looks very pleased, saying something like "beautiful view," and we move on to the bathroom. There, I explain that there's also a separate toilet. And then we enter the sun-drenched living room with kitchen.

Tatjana holds the baby in her arms and seems thoroughly delighted. The anticipation of a great vacation is practically written all over her face.

Sergej, on the other hand, is already looking for the first flaws before he's even seen the highlight of the vacation rental. The three hundred fifty-five square feet terrace with a sea view. I can tell from his face, even as I keep smiling.

"Baby sleep?" he asks accusingly, pointing to his son in Tatjana's arms.

"In the bedroom," I reply even more cheerfully, thinking: The crib in the bedroom was hard to miss. Well, then let's go together to the bedroom with the sea view and the baby bed, I decide. Then Sergej can have another look.

Unfortunately, things don't improve with Sergej in the coming days. He incessantly calls my name, summoning me upstairs to the vacation rental to ask seemingly trivial questions.

I can't shake the feeling that he's determined to assert his authority over me. However, he hasn't anticipated my emancipated reluctance to follow his instructions. While that may work at his home, we'll need to figure out a different arrangement here, I think irritably in such moments.

But I wisely keep my mouth shut. There must be a strategy to put our dear guest in his place without offending him.

Yet after a few days, I can't stand Sergej's voice anymore. Every time he calls my name, I flinch.

More out of anger than fear, I explain to my mother, who's already quite concerned.

"That can't be good for the baby," she says.

That's the thing about guests. They pay for a nice vacation, and they should get it. But not at any cost, I always say. So it's time for Sergej to understand that too. And in a twist of fate, the chance to make that clear to him has arrived when he once again summons me upstairs.

'What does he want this time?' I think, feeling the heat rising inside me. You need to calm down. He's our guest, I keep repeating to myself as I walk through the garden and then up the stairs to the vacation rental.

It's hot, and I'm sweating like after a marathon. And that's just the beginning of the pregnancy, I think as I arrive upstairs and take a deep breath.

Now you'll ring the bell and walk back down two steps so you don't end up sticking to his thick, naked belly, I think to myself.

Because that's how he's been presenting himself for the past few days. And once again, Sergej, dressed only in swim trunks, opens the door to the vacation rental and smirks when he sees me.

Shortly after, Tatjana appears behind him in the doorway, holding the baby, looking unsure.

"You iron," Sergej says, grinning and pointing his finger at me.

"Excuse me?" I ask irritably, even though I know exactly what he means. He wants me to iron for him! He's lost his mind, I think angrily, wiping beads of sweat from my upper lip.

"You don't have iron," he changes tactics when he seems to notice my rising anger.

Yes, we do have iron, I think, wanting to explain to him that we do indeed have an iron and an ironing board in one of the bedrooms for him. But then his wife Tatjana interrupts our conversation.

"We have, Sergej, we have iron," she tries to explain to him meekly. But he talks over her, waving his arm backward, telling her to be quiet.

"No. You iron," he now asserts more firmly, pointing at me once again.

This can't be real, I think angrily. He knows they have an iron available. And yet he insists that I iron for him just because he's the guest. And a Russian guest at that.

But suddenly, a warm feeling washes over me, and I hear myself smiling and mimicking his accent as I reply: "I hate iron."

Forget it, Sergej, I hate ironing, and that won't change in the next forty-one days you're still here.

Tatjana freezes in shock, Sergej looks at me in disbelief. I just stand there and smile, and gradually Sergej seems to actually understand that you shouldn't mess with the sweating, hormone-flooded host.

In the second week of June, Mia calls me from the city. At first, she tells me in detail about another date with her colleague Ben. She seems happy, but after a few minutes, I sense that something is bothering her, so I ask.

Yes, there's something else she needs to tell me. She wanted to keep it to herself until she arrived on the island with us. But now she can't wait any longer.

While studying for the upcoming exams at university, she noticed that she couldn't hold the highlighter with her right hand, she tells me worriedly. Also, her right arm keeps getting numb, which is quite annoying. Especially since she needs enough time to prepare properly for the exams. She asks me what she should do now.

Actually, there's an ultrasound scheduled in the next few days, for which Tony and I planned to go to the mainland, but now we'll have to change our plans.

I'm concerned and don't want to leave Mia alone with her worries. So, we drive back home to the city and combine a visit to Doctor Harper with the ultrasound at my gynecologist's office.

Just two days later, we're in Doctor Harper's examination room. He doesn't seem concerned and starts by asking Mia if she's stressed about exams.

"Not really," she replies. "I enjoy studying."

"Nevertheless, any kind of stress isn't good for you, Mia. You know that. Take it to heart while studying," he advises her with a smile.

Then, turning to me, he adds, "Right now, I wouldn't want to administer corticosteroids. The next treatment with the medication is scheduled for early August, and she'll receive corticosteroids then too. That would be too close together for my liking. So, let's wait it out. It'll go away on its own once she relaxes a bit."

And indeed, somewhat reassured by his words, I sit in my gynecologist's waiting room the next day with Tony.

Today is June 13th, I remember. St. Anthony's Day. Tony's name day. I can't think of a better gift than hearing the baby's first heartbeat, I think to myself, smiling as I observe the other waiting couples. If they only knew how old I am, and pregnant on top of it, I think proudly.

After an hour of waiting, my gynecologist asks me into his examination room.

"I'll go in alone first, then he'll fetch you when it's time," I explain to Tony, giving him a kiss on the cheek.

"Hmm, your blood pressure is a bit elevated," Doctor Johnson informs me as he removes the blood pressure cuff from my arm a few minutes later.

"The excitement," I reply. No wonder, I add in my thoughts, this is all so exciting.

"Well, the expectant dad must be proud, right? He can come in when we're ready," he smiles, and I settle onto the examination table.

Uncomfortable things, these tables, I think, as Doctor Johnson tries to locate the embryo on the ultrasound screen.

"Can you see anything yet?" I ask excitedly.

"Yes, I can see something already. But now, let's check the heartbeat. You're in your ninth week, and the dad surely wants to hear something, doesn't he?"

"I'm sure he's pacing in the hallway already because he can't wait," I explain, laughing, but Doctor Johnson suddenly looks concerned.

Quiet and focused, he seems to be searching for the heartbeat and turns up the volume on the machine.

Minutes pass as I lie on the examination table, staring at the ceiling, waiting. Waiting for a sound, a reassuring word from Doctor Johnson.

And finally, there's a clear sound coming from the ultrasound machine. I exhale in relief.

"Well, there's something," I hear myself say. But his expression freezes me the next moment.

Once again, he turns up the volume, apparently listening for a sound.

"Those are just the sounds of your blood vessels," he explains almost silently and looks at me. "Unfortunately, not the sounds of the heart," he adds. "There's nothing. I'm sorry."

The room falls into a hushed stillness. There I lay, coming to terms with the inevitable truth—it is over once more. The anticipation, the dreams, the hopes, and that fleeting moment of joy that embraced us—all of it now slipping through our fingers once again.

A week later, Tony and I find ourselves in Doctor Johnson's waiting room at seven in the morning. I stare at my sun-kissed legs and the deep blue summer dress. I would have worn this dress more often in the future to conceal my growing belly.

It's a favorite of mine, but maybe I should retire it to the closet after today, I think as we wait.

Besides us, there's only a young couple in the gynecologist's office this morning.

I wonder why the young woman is here at this hour. Maybe she's experiencing a miscarriage too. Or something else. She's not ready for the baby. She's young, and the timing might not be right. Or maybe I'm wrong. She seems anxious, whispering to her partner constantly.

Shortly after, Doctor Johnson calls Sara into the examination room. So that's her name. Sara.

When she emerges from the examination room about ten minutes later, she looks very pale.

A nurse escorts her and her partner to the elevator, and then it's my turn.

About twenty minutes later, I spot Sara again. We're both sharing a patient room.

A nice room with a view of the city, I think as I settle onto the bed by the window.

The nurse asks if we want a privacy screen between the beds. I decline, glancing over at Sara. She seems to be in pain, curled up on her bed, shaking her head.

Well, it seems she got the pill instead of a procedure, just like me, I think as I sit cross-legged on the bed.

Wearing a dress today wasn't such a great idea after all. I should have thought about that. But right now, I don't really care. After all, we're both women, and in this situation, we're already exposed to each other.

I gaze out the window, reflecting on the past week. After Doctor Johnson confirmed a week ago that there was no heartbeat on the ultrasound machine, we had to discuss the next steps. Brief and matter-of-fact.

If I were to consider another pregnancy at my age, he advised against a curettage procedure. The tissue would be too severely injured and would scar afterward.

That sounded reasonable, so I opted for the second option. Tablets that would induce the embryo to be expelled from my body.

Even the mere thought, now that I'm actually sitting on this bed in the hospital, is dreadful. After all, the baby was supposed to grow, not be expelled and flushed down the toilet.

I won't dwell on how all of this will happen, I admonish myself. And I won't envision any of it in detail or let images form in my mind, I think, glancing over at Sara.

By now, she seems to be in severe pain. She's curled up in bed, facing the wall.

After about fifteen minutes, I know how she feels because I feel it myself. The tablets are taking effect, and it dawns on me what's happening here.

These pains are very familiar to me. Labor-like contractions every five minutes, pushing everything forward.

After some time, Sara can't take it anymore and tearfully asks the nurse for a painkiller. Once she's calmed down a bit, she turns to me.

"Is it as bad for you?" she asks hesitantly.

"Yes, but I'm a bit older than you. I know these pains from giving birth to my daughter," I reply. "It'll pass, then you'll feel better."

"My mother doesn't know," she then confides, bursting into tears again. "I'm in the middle of my dental studies. How am I supposed to manage that? My boyfriend wanted us to keep it, but that would be too much for me," she tries to explain.

She needs to tell someone, I think to myself, and she can tell me. After all, I could be her mother.

"You know, my daughter is about your age. You're still young. When the time comes, you'll have a baby. There's no point in blaming yourself," I console her.

But secretly, it hits me hard that I had wanted the baby and now feel cheated. She, on the other hand, could have kept it but chooses not to. That's life, I sadly conclude.

Yet, I don't really want to fully embrace the emotions surging within me about the lost baby. I have to keep functioning. Mia needs me.

"And you?" Sara asks, pulling me out of my thoughts.

"Well," I begin, without looking at her. "I'm almost forty-four. The little heart didn't beat. Maybe it'll work out another time," I try to keep my story brief.

I can see what she's thinking. That she feels ashamed for what she decided and ended prematurely. That's why I change the subject.

"Actually, I should be somewhere else today. My daughter Mia has her second exam at university today, and I should be helping her with her writing. She has MS and can't hold a pen at the moment," I explain to Sara, checking my watch. It's already eight. Surely Mia and Tony have already left for the university.

"A friend of mine also has MS. I have a number I can give you. There's this guy who's into herbal remedies. My friend says it helps very well."

"Yeah, that would be nice," I reply, even though my mind is elsewhere. I imagine Mia sitting in the car, nervously going over the material in her head again.

Mrs. Angel will be writing the exam for Mia today. How it came about still surprises me.

Shortly after confirming today's appointment, I called her and explained that I had a hospital procedure that couldn't be rescheduled.

What else could I have said?

Tony offered to take the exam with Mia. I asked Mrs. Angel if that would work, but she had already made her decision by then.

She would do it, she said. At that hour, she had no supervision and would be in her office, she explained.

Whether that's really the case, I don't know, but I am touched by this gesture.

Mia is equally surprised. A woman like Mrs. Angel, who doesn't tolerate distractions during her lectures and demands full attention, offers her support.

Mia often tells me that Mrs. Angel always checks during lecture what knowledge from the previous lecture has stuck. You always have to be prepared for her further questions.

However, she always advocates for her students. She's one of the few professors who remains approachable and hasn't distanced herself from the reason for her work: the students.

Mia hasn't told any of her classmates that Mrs. Angel will be writing down the exam for her.

Why invite unnecessary gossip? It benefits no one if they find out and potentially draw the wrong conclusions.

Two hours later, Sara has fallen asleep. I lie in bed and stare at the ceiling of the patient room. It's quiet, and I feel somewhat dazed from the pain, which is finally behind me. The sun streams into the room, and I hear the traffic from outside.

Why does all this have to happen, I wonder as I lie here. Can't life just be easy? At some point, it has to be sufficient. First, dealing with Mia's situation, then the miscarriage.

Next week, we'll head back to the island, and I'll have to deal with the guests once more. Being polite, cleaning, suppressing emotions. Not showing what I really think.

If only I could get out of all this crap. Doing something that's truly amazing. Something I've been dreaming about for so long.

Why do we keep putting things off, I ask myself the next moment. We're so careless. We think we can always do it later. But can we really?

The Camino de Santiago would be nice, I think then. Mia and I have been planning that for a long time. Camino de Santiago in five-star style, we always joke. We'd do it differently from everyone else. A pilgrimage in luxury and yet with enlightenment.

With or without makeup is one of the questions we often ask ourselves when discussing the seemingly fundamental aspects of such a journey. Because if you want to post photos along the way, you still want to look good despite all the hardships, we think.

However, a pilgrimage of at least three weeks requires extensive preparation. The minimum of three hundred kilometers is indeed a considerable distance. And long walks are probably not feasible at the moment. Who knows when something will happen with her leg again. We certainly don't want to get stuck in the middle of the journey.

But we could fly, it occurs to me. How about London? That's been Mia's dream destination since high school.

For the first time that day, I smile as I imagine the two of us admiring Big Ben or standing in front of the guards at Buckingham Palace.

Mia will make faces to make the guards laugh. No one would expect a perfectly put-together young woman to be ready to act silly here. But that's just her.

So, we're going to London, I whisper, as if my spoken words would make this plan come true.

And the quiet excitement about it almost makes me feel something like happiness in that moment.

Ten days have passed since my visit to the gynecologist's office, and we're back on the island. The abrupt hormonal change still makes me keenly aware that life doesn't just go on as if nothing had happened.

Every night, I dream about the baby. Most of the time, it's a boy I'm holding in my arms. Sometimes, it's a girl. I call them by their name and stroke their soft baby skin.

When I wake up, all I feel is emptiness. Once again, I've failed. I couldn't carry the baby to term.

Once again, I couldn't give Tony his own child, Mia a sibling, and my mother a second grandchild.

Tony doesn't talk much about what happened. He seems different when we're together. I'm afraid this loss might come between us. Unspoken but present.

Perhaps he unconsciously blames me, thinking it's my fault we don't have a child together.

But then I redirect my thoughts to the day ahead and push all that aside. After all, life must go on. Life holds other things in store for us, I think to myself. And I console myself with the excitement of my travel plans and the upcoming surprise.

Just a few days ago, I spontaneously booked two flights to London.

For September, because in August, we have the second round of treatment with the medication. After that, we can safely travel, and by then, Mia can recover. Her arm will surely be fine by then too.

Plus, we want to go to London during a season when everything is still green. That way, we can stroll through the famous Hyde Park and inhale the scent of nature. Right in the heart of the city.

"We're flying on September 17th and staying for five days," I surprised Mia a few days after booking. "Are you excited?"

She was lying in her bed in the afternoon, experiencing pain in her arm.

"I can hardly believe it," she replied, and I could see the joy in her eyes.

"You really booked it already? Then we'll celebrate your birthday in London."

"Yeah, I know. My forty-fourth. The flights are booked. Now we just need to pick a hotel. I didn't want to do that without you."

We decided on a boutique hotel with only sixteen rooms in a Georgian townhouse on the same day. Four stars in the trendy neighborhood of Marylebone, where we might bump into Madonna and other stars on the sidewalk because they live around there. Quite expensive, but special.

We want to feel like we're in an old British TV series. In my mind, I can already hear the horse-drawn carriage pulling up. Two ladies occupy the fireplace room on the first floor. Breakfast will be served downstairs in the salon from eight to ten in the morning. Then the day's program begins with culture and music. In the afternoon, tea time with cake snacks is planned, and in the evening, international specialties will be served in one of the nearby restaurants.

All of this away from the hotel bustle, in a quiet, elegant atmosphere. At least that's how we envision our stay in London.

Well, the overnight rate for this British delight initially shocked me. But fortunately, Sergej has been a guest in our vacation home long enough to financially enable us to pursue this dream. A dream that is soon to come true.

July 2017

I'm starting to get impatient. The Neurology Day Clinic still hasn't given us a date for the second treatment with the medication.

By mid-July, I can't take it anymore, so I call the clinic. The receptionist tells me there's an issue with the treatment authorization from the clinic's end. Doctor Harper has signed all the documents, but the final signature from the clinic's management is missing.

"How am I supposed to understand this?" I ask, getting agitated. "Mia received the first cycle, and now it's supposed to stop there? The medication only kicks in after the second dose." I take several deep breaths to keep from yelling at the lady on the phone. "Please connect me to Doctor Harper. This can't be happening."

When he finally answers after several rings, I don't even know where to begin.

"Doctor Harper, the receptionist just told me that Mia isn't getting the second dose of the medication. Is that true?"

"Well, we had scheduled the treatment for early August. However, the clinic management doesn't want to sign off on the treatment authorization because Mia had a rash after the first cycle," he explains.

"That's true, but it disappeared after a day," I interject. "And isn't that listed as a common side effect? That's what the official leaflet says. I've thoroughly researched everything online."

"You're right. However, the clinic doesn't want to take any risks if a patient reacts to the medication like that. After all, there could be more serious side effects," he responds.

"But I don't understand. Couldn't they have said something earlier? It's been a year since the first treatment. That's quite a revelation for the clinic management," I respond, feeling the anger rise within me, and I have to repeatedly remind myself to stay calm.

"You know, things work a bit differently here," he explains. "The clinic management only reviews the treatment records when a signature is required. And that's only happening now, after a year," he responds and his voice sounds reserved.

"Do you think Mia won't get the second treatment?" I ask, feeling my pulse quicken at the thought.

"I can't make any promises, unfortunately. The clinic management has the final say," he explains. "But don't worry for now. I'll try to sort this out," he adds. But his words don't calm me at that moment.

"You know, Doctor Harper, we understand that this medication isn't just beneficial for Mia's body, but it also harms her in a way. So I don't understand why the clinic management even considers just cutting Mia off with an incomplete treatment. I mean, ultimately, she gains nothing from the medication after just one dose, and yet the damage is still done. They know the long-term effects of the medication," I express my concerns.

"I completely understand your worries, and I know you're concerned about Mia," he responds, pausing briefly. It sounds like he's taking notes as we talk. "In the next few days, I have another meeting with the clinic management, then we'll see," he assures me.

"And what if the clinic management doesn't approve the treatment?"

"This medication is currently the most advanced on the market," he answers, hesitating. "Unfortunately, another treatment isn't an option for this aggressive form of MS."

August 2017

Meanwhile, it's already August, and we're right in the middle of the rental season. Since last week, a Swiss couple in their early thirties and their two school-age boys have been staying in our vacation rental.

They're not particularly talkative. They prefer to only crack the door to the vacation rental a bit when I ring the bell to bring fresh towels.

I understand, though. I'd probably do the same if I were the guest. Reserved yet friendly. After all, you want your vacation to be spent alone, not with the host.

Anyway, I don't let these things bother me anymore; I'm busy preparing for our trip to London.

There are organizational matters to take care of, things I need to plan ahead for. Like, for instance, what to do about the guests in the house? Because at the beginning of September, my mother will leave the island and go back home. Then there won't be anyone in the house to check on the guests.

"Don't worry," I try to calm her down. "Just before we leave, our Scottish guests will arrive. Mavis and her husband. They're both over sixty. She wants to paint the untouched nature and the village. That doesn't sound to me like they'll be throwing wild parties in our vacation rental," I add.

My mother doesn't seem completely reassured, but to me, it sounds like a couple who just wants to relax in peace. And guests like that can safely be left alone in the house.

Besides, Tony promised me to drop by the house occasionally, just to check in. Of course, it'll be under some pretext. He'll just ring the doorbell and ask the guests if they need anything. Towels, wine, or even some advice.

That way, my mother's concerns will be completely eased, and Mia and I can enjoy our trip in peace.

Days pass by, and still, no one from the clinic has called. Mia spends a lot of time with her friends and seems content. Almost daily, she heads to the beach with them in the late afternoon and to the café in the evenings.

Yet, I can see her worry about what might happen if she doesn't get the medication anymore.

Every now and then I catch a glimpse of her worried face when she feels unobserved. I can see her obviously contemplating the possibility of the second treatment being denied.

But when I bring it up, she brushes it off. She's not worried, she reassures me repeatedly. So far, she is doing okay.

However, I can't quite believe her. I doubt her supposed nonchalance. She's probably just grappling with it internally, I think.

So, we hardly raise the issue. Occasionally, Mia asks casually if the clinic has called. After lunch or in passing. No, they haven't, is all I can reply. And then we move on to daily matters as if nothing had happened.

It seems like she doesn't want to place too much significance on that question. It's as if she's trying, through this casualness, to keep open the possibility of living a life without the medication. Trying to avoid becoming dependent on it.

Meanwhile, the thought of the clinic possibly rejecting the second treatment has weighed heavily on me in recent days, to the point where I can't fall asleep at night.

Scenarios of her future keep swirling in my mind, contemplating how far the disease could progress without proper treatment. What options would remain for us. And how we could obtain the medication ourselves if needed.

At night, I lie awake in bed, and Doctor Harper's last words keep echoing in my mind: "Another treatment isn't an option for Mia. It's an aggressive form of MS."

Currently, she's doing well. She's walking, able to use her hands. But what if that changes? That question pushes all my past wishes and plans for her into the background. Suddenly, all my visions of a happy and carefree future for her seem to have been pushed far into the distance.

I wonder if we now have to live in constant fear that a new relapse could occur. An even more devastating one. One from which she may not recover.

As I lie awake at night, all the dreadful experiences people describe on their accounts on the internet come to mind. In forums, those patients describe relapses where the symptoms didn't regress. Now, they're bound to wheelchairs. They can't eat, bathe, let alone leave the house on their own. A life dependent on others. Without freedom and without hope of improvement.

What will I do if it comes to that, I ask myself on nights like these. How will life go on for us then?

Our upcoming trip to London is my only bright spot these days. Constantly, I scour the internet for what we could see there. Which museums we shouldn't miss and where we can find the best restaurants on our day trips through the British metropolis.

Every day is meant to be a highlight. Everything is scheduled from morning after breakfast in the hotel to bedtime late in the evening.

Some time ago, I created a special Excel spreadsheet for our trip. Everything is carefully planned and color-coded.

From Notting Hill to a "Jesus Christ Superstar" musical in Regent's Park, to a walking tour through the nocturnal London on the paths of the most famous serial killers. We want to experience it all. In time lapse, as if there's no tomorrow.

Furthermore, I meticulously record every subway route from point A to B, along with their exact travel times, in the spreadsheet. This way, we don't waste any unnecessary time during our explorations of London.

Of course, I'm being a bit too meticulous. However, we never want to find ourselves standing in front of a museum or church in London without knowing where the nearest bus or train goes.

But a few days before our departure, I delete the subway routes from my Excel spreadsheet when an attack on the London Underground makes the news. We opt for the bus instead.

So, I look up all the bus routes with their schedules and enter them instead of the subway rides. The rides might take longer, but at least we'll get to see more of the city.

Plus, we decide to avoid the London Bridge after the recent events.

"It's bad enough that I have MS. I'd like us to experience our trip to London from start to finish. It would be a shame with all the money you're spending," Mia explains, laughing.

"Well, we can't exactly demand a refund if we end up dead in a ditch," I reply, laughing at our inside joke.

As I sit in front of my laptop again at the end of August, looking at our Excel spreadsheet, it hits me for the first time. Soon, we'll actually experience everything that's been written in that Excel spreadsheet on my laptop. And for a brief moment, that makes me happy.

September 2017

Ten days later, I receive a call from Doctor Harper.

"I think we've done it," he explains. "The clinic management is ready to sign the treatment authorization next week."

"Is that certain?" I ask. "I mean, why didn't they sign right away? It sounds like they might change their minds," I add.

"Well, we had a clinic meeting yesterday. I presented Mia's case and made it clear to the management that she urgently needs the second dose due to the advanced lesions," he responds.

"And what did they say? Was the rash discussed?" I ask, feeling impatient.

"Yes, that issue was raised, and I believe I managed to address their concerns," he explains.

"So, she'll definitely get the second dose?"

There's a brief, almost imperceptible hesitation in his voice.

"That's what I was assured of yesterday," he replies. "Let's wait until next week. I'll contact you as soon as I have the signature," he concludes the call.

What remains is a feeling caught between budding joy and anxious restraint.

Nothing's certain in this life, I think for the umpteenth time in that moment.

Two days before our departure, I'm busy measuring our suitcases to check if they qualify as carry-on luggage when I receive a text message:

Confirming your appointment on 09/25/2017 at 8 AM at the Neurology Day Clinic, it reads. It takes me a few seconds to realize that this must be about the appointment for the second treatment dose.

Shortly after, the head nurse from the Neurology Day Clinic calls me to make sure I received the automated appointment confirmation via SMS.

So, the clinic management has signed off, I think, barely able to contain my excitement.

Finally, life can move forward. And finally, there's hope for a normal life. For a life without fear. Even far into the future.

– Chapter 6 –

September 17, 2017

The day has come. At eleven o'clock, Mia and I are on the plane to London, and our long-planned trip can begin.

Over the next five days, we'll forget about MS and enjoy life as only the two of us can.

We toast with champagne and wave out the window like royalty as the plane takes off. Mia quickly takes selfies that she wants to post later. No moment should go by without capturing it for her followers.

The legroom in first class is excellent, and with the glossy magazines provided, time will literally fly by.

At least, that's how we feel. The reality, however, is quite different. The plane is actually pretty cramped, especially since it's fully packed, and the budget airline doesn't even offer complimentary water.

Mia snagged a window seat on my left, while on my right, there's an overweight, middle-aged man with a receding hairline, engrossed in his sports newspaper.

There's not much room to maneuver, but the destination makes it all worthwhile.

Over the next few hours, I'll try to suppress my claustrophobia and mentally focus on the Excel spreadsheet in my suitcase.

However, a few minutes into the flight, unexpected turbulence sets in. The plane sways back and forth.

My expression must look so panicked that Mia tells me to calm down.

I clutch the armrests. She, on the other hand, sits calmly and seems unfazed.

A thousand thoughts race through my mind. We're going to die. On the flight to the city of her dreams. I had everything planned so perfectly. The budget flight, the ridiculously expensive hotel. And now this.

It's my fault. We're going to crash, and it's my fault. If only we had stayed home. Screw this trip! First MS, and now we're going to die too.

After a few minutes, when the turbulence subsides and calm returns to the plane, I take a deep breath and glance around. No one seems to have noticed my panic.

Mia smiles at me, and I feel a bit foolish.

"You know, it's just my flight anxiety," I whisper, settling back into my seat, trying to act like nothing can bother me. "Anyway, when we get there, I'm going to need a doughnut," I add, reclining in my seat.

Because in London, we've decided to ignore our good intentions about diet for five days. Away from MS and inflammation-free diets, we've decided to live like ordinary folks.

After all, Mia is doing well, and sometimes you just have to indulge in life's culinary pleasures. With sugary treats and all the trimmings.

And they're already within reach as we land at Gatwick a few hours later, a bit delayed. Finally, we breathe in London air.

Now nothing can go wrong, and our five-day adventure begins.

September 18, 2017

My forty-fourth birthday begins at six in the morning when my phone alarm goes off. Mia is still asleep. She was cold last night and seemed exhausted from the journey. So, I turned the heat up on the air conditioning in the evening and left it running all night to keep her warm and prevent her from catching a cold.

As I glance at my phone screen, I take a screenshot to capture this day and this moment. It's September 18, 2017, at 6:13 a.m. in London.

The weather app says it's going to be around sixty-four degrees today, and it's expected to stay dry, which is unusual for London this time of year.

Well, that sounds like a nice start to our London adventure.

And about two hours later, on this sunny day, after a hearty hotel breakfast, our first item on the agenda awaits us.

Notting Hill. Following in the footsteps of Julia Roberts and Hugh Grant. What else? Even if the Portobello Road seems much smaller than in the movie, that doesn't diminish our enthusiasm for actually being here.

It's pretty crowded here too.

We expected the famous street to be popular as a backdrop. But we didn't expect so many tourists to be out this early in the morning.

Everywhere, mostly young women, but also others, are obviously posing for the perfect Notting Hill photo for their social media followers.

An artificial smile here, a seemingly natural and entirely random walking motion there.

"Who knows how many times she'll have to repeat that 'natural' stride today," I comment as we pass by.

"At least the lighting's good," Mia replies, and we grin at each other. "We need to take a few photos of me too so I can post them tonight," she adds.

So, I take photos of Mia. Instead of the clearly professional cameras that others have, I only have my phone. But she thinks that should suffice.

Occasionally, I also capture a snapshot of Mia just for myself. Like when her long, golden-brown hair cascades over her shoulders as she looks at a silver ring at a jewelry stand. A smile, visible only to me, plays at the corners of her mouth.

These fleeting moments I want to capture in photos for myself, to remember them later.

To remind myself what her happiness looks like through my eyes.

"Do you like the ring?" I ask her.

"Yes, it's really nice with that turquoise stone," she replies, visibly taken with it.

"Then let's get it as a souvenir from London," I decide.

Who could refuse her this wish, I think for the rest of the day, as she admires the ring on her finger over and over again.

September 19, 2017

Early in the morning, right after breakfast, we take a bus to the university city of Oxford. It's a must-see, I thought, when I added this stop to our itinerary before our trip.

First, we visit the city's main library, the Bodleian Library, with a guided tour. We didn't know it also served as a backdrop for the Harry Potter movies. And that wasn't our reason for coming here. Nevertheless, we find it fascinating to learn about the history of the library and a bit about filming in these halls. A young tour guide explains how each book spine had to be covered specifically for the film scenes.

As long as it's about books, everything is interesting, I think to myself. Because we love books. So, when visiting Oxford, a library must naturally be part of the program.

When we subsequently visit a Jane Austen exhibition, Mia makes an unexpected discovery. Alongside the author's handwritten notes, there's a volume describing a nerve condition in one of the display cases.

"Not even here can I escape it," she remarks, and I feel how this brief moment of our trip adds a bitter undertone.

But on the journey back to London, those thoughts have long dissipated. The anticipation of our evening highlight overshadows everything else.

Andrew Lloyd Webber's masterpiece, the musical "Jesus Christ Superstar," is being performed tonight in the open-air theater of Regent's Park. A unique spectacle under the London night sky. And we're part of it. In two very expensive, but also very good seats.

But it's worth it to us. So, we spend the late afternoon before the musical in the hotel room, indulging in tea-time and doughnuts on the king size bed.

And just before eight o'clock, we finally take our seats in the packed audience stands at Regent's Park. It's almost dark already, with the birds singing their evening hymns into the sky.

This performance is one of the most beautiful experiences of my life, I think, as the lead actress sings the song of Mary Magdalene an hour later.

Her words touch me deeply, and tears stream down my cheeks.

In that moment, I feel both the happiness and sorrow of life, with its countless twists and turns.

A life that fulfills our desires in one moment and devastates our hopes for a bright tomorrow in the next.

Yet, despite it all, I am happy. Happy that we're here. My sweetie and I. My everything.

I am happy that I could fulfill her long-held wish for this trip. Not postponing it like so many other things.

But, I wonder now, would I have done the same if she hadn't been diagnosed with MS. Probably not. Not at this moment.

Other things would have been more important. The university, the work, my company.

"Isn't this amazing?" Mia asks when she sees my tears.

"Yes, simply indescribable," I reply. I smile at her. "I love you, sweetie." And you don't have to be afraid, I add silently. I'll always be with you. No matter what.

September 20, 2017

Today is Mia's day. She's chosen the day's itinerary. In the late morning, we take the bus to Hyde Park to see where the British royal family resides.

"Damn, we've caught the Changing of the Guard," I remark as we arrive at Buckingham Palace.

"Guess I can forget about making faces at the guards. That would've been such a good photo op," Mia responds.

Nevertheless, we take photos of the guards, the police horses, and manage to convince a handsome policeman to take a photo with Mia.

"That's a wrap," I declare as we then make our way back to the bus, "we've got that in the can."

"Well, the palace isn't particularly grand. I imagined it much bigger," Mia comments.

"Anyway, at least we were there and got to see it."

"You know what, Mom. Let's deviate from our plan today and go to the Tower of London. We were supposed to avoid that part of the city, but I'd like to see it," she suggests as we're about to board the bus to Covent Garden.

"Why not? Let's do it. Let me just quickly find the bus route on my map," I reply. "I wasn't prepared for that," I add, and we both laugh at how it momentarily throws me off.

Two hours later, we've thoroughly explored the area around the Tower of London and are heading towards Big Ben. Originally, we planned to take the bus there, as noted on my list. But Mia wants a boat ride on the Thames. So off we go to the ticket counter. The day is rainy and windy, just as one would expect from London. Yet one thing mustn't be missed.

"Now we just need to snap a photo of you with the bridge in the background. That screams London," I suggest as we walk to the ferry.

Apparently, we're not the only ones with this idea, as there seems to be a line here to get a photo with the bridge in the background.

But the wait is worth it.

"This is perfect," Mia declares as she sees the photo on her phone. "I absolutely have to post this later."

Half an hour later, the ferry docks near Big Ben. Shrouded in scaffolding but still recognizable, it towers into the sky.

"You know what, we could continue with one of those rickshaws. That could be fun," I suggest when I spot a few of them on a platform in front of Big Ben.

"Cool. Are you sure it's not too expensive?" Mia asks.

"Even if it is. We're in London. The sign says twenty pounds, but I'll double-check with the driver," I reply.

"Twenty pounds to Oxford Street," he explains in an Eastern European accent.

"Let's do it," I tell Mia, and we hop in. However, what happens next catches us off guard. We zoom through the honking London rush hour traffic in what feels like thirty seconds. The wind whips through our hair, and I fear we might fall out of the rickshaw at this speed. After all, we're not strapped in.

"This is pretty fast," I shout to the driver up front, but he seems to ignore my concern and keeps speeding ahead.

Meanwhile, Mia is thoroughly amused and snaps photos of everything she can. And I capture her joy.

Chinatown blurs past us. I only catch glimpses of red lanterns and Chinese characters. That's my only indication that we've just passed through this neighborhood.

And before we know it, we've arrived at Oxford Street.

We haven't even fully gotten out when the driver demands forty pounds.

Surprised by this sudden price change, I try to explain to him that he had announced twenty pounds earlier.

"Per person," he says, and his tone becomes unpleasant. He keeps looking around nervously.

Somehow, I find this ridiculous, but his harsh tone leaves no room for discussion. He wants forty pounds, end of story.

So, I pay him.

"This can't be real," I mutter after he finally speeds off. Angry at my own gullibility, I shake my head.

"But it was still funny," Mia remarks, grinning.

"True, and we won't forget this ride anytime soon.

But… let's head to the hotel now. I need a cup of tea to calm down."

After resting at the hotel until late afternoon, we finally embark on Mia's highlight of this trip: the "Blood and Tears Walk" through nocturnal London.

It's almost dark when we arrive at the Barbican subway station around seven in the evening. This is where we meet up with an actor who will guide us on the trail of past serial killers.

For two hours, we walk through London's dimly lit streets with a group of about ten people, eagerly listening to his captivating stories that go beyond just the tales of Jack the Ripper.

We stop beside a cemetery in the middle of the city. It's dark, and he tells us how gravediggers used to smuggle fresh corpses to the nearby hospital for payment right here. "The doctors needed real human bodies," he explains, "to learn what they previously only knew from animal carcasses."

It's pretty creepy standing here in the dark and imagining all of that. But it's definitely intriguing.

Shortly after, in London's financial district, he tells us about a particularly bizarre murder. One evening many years ago, a tourist visited one of the local bars. There, he met a London bank employee who wanted to have a beer after work.

The Londoner seemed to find the tourist so nice that he invited him to his home.

The next day, the tourist was found dead on the bank employee's couch. With headphones still playing music.

It was said the bank employee just needed some company.

With these stories, we finally head back to the hotel around nine o'clock via the subway.

Along the way, we grab a bucket of chicken wings for our hotel "home". Arriving in our hotel room, we get comfy in our pajamas on the bed. But with the bucket still half full, we can't eat another bite.

"What do we do with the rest? It's like the smell's wafting down to reception," I ask Mia, scanning the room. "And the trash can is out of the question," I add.

"Maybe there's a trash bin down on the street," Mia suggests.

But when I try to open the window, I'm disappointed.

"I guess they're keen on keeping the suicide rate low here," I remark, struggling with the window. "It only opens halfway."

"Well, forget that. Now what?" Mia asks. "I suggest we grab some bags and…" I say, pointing to the closet.

" … the chicken wings will have to sleep in the closet," Mia adds with a grin.

And the idea of chicken wings spending the night in the closet has us in tears of laughter.

Typical Mia and me, I think later that evening as we're already in bed.

And typical girls, always finding a way, no matter what.

December 2017

London is now two months behind us. Right after returning, I bid farewell to our last holiday guests, Mavis and Albert, on the island, and officially declared the rental season over for the year.

Then it was back home. Back to our city life.

Just the three of us. Tony, Mia and me. Without guests' wishes. Without constantly being called or bombarded with text messages asking trivial questions that I'd rather not answer.

Only a few days after our arrival in the city, Mia received the second dose of the medication. Since then, she's been doing excellent. She's back to her routine at the university. Lectures and meetings with classmates fill her schedule. Just an ordinary student life.

However, there's something new in her life.

Since early October, she and Ben have been a couple. She seems happy. Yet, I can't help but feel skeptical whenever she talks about him. Currently, he doesn't want a serious relationship, as he casually mentioned to her. He needs his space. Nevertheless, they're still together.

Her expression subtly changes as she tells me about it one evening. She's sitting at her vanity, combing her hair. But she keeps pausing, looking pensive. It hurts her, I think, and I want to comfort her. Still, she insists they're happy, and he didn't mean it that way, she explains, as if she could read my mind. That's not the Mia I know. That's not the Mia who knows who she is and always follows her own rules. Especially in a relationship.

However, this time everything's different, and I'm starting to understand what the reason for that might be.

Towards the end of November, I increasingly witness Mia sitting at home, waiting long past the agreed time for her appointments with Ben. I wonder about this behavior but say nothing. Tony never did this to me. Just leaving me sitting and waiting like that. I find it disrespectful. But I stay silent. Mia tells me that something always comes up for him, apparently without blaming him for it. He's just really busy with university, the gym, and casting calls for commercials, she says.

They book him for commercials and billboard ads. Anyway, he's always on the go. Meanwhile, I wonder why he keeps making plans with her on days when he won't have time anyway. It's always like, he'll let her know if he can make it to the appointment. Or rather, if he can't, I add in my thoughts. He wants to string her along. Be the one calling the shots. But I wonder why? Is it his silent realization that she's grateful to have found someone? Despite her illness. This thought haunts me, and suspicion starts to grow.

So, I decide to keep an eye on this Ben from now on.

"Ben and I are planning to go away for New Year's," Mia tells us one evening in early December during dinner. "It doesn't matter where. Just away. I've already picked out a few nearby destinations," she adds.

"Well, a change of scenery can only do you good," Tony responds, looking pleased.

I, on the other hand, am not thrilled, but I keep quiet. Lately, I've seen her coming home in the evenings and heard her crying in the bathroom shortly after.

She doesn't talk about it, and I try to hold back, though I know something has been off in their relationship for a while. Sometimes she seems elated when she meets up with him. On other days, she seems deeply hurt. His inconsistent behavior is obviously the reason for this. Sometimes he picks her up from university every day, and they post photos together—whether in the cafeteria during lunch, on a walk, or at the movies. Then, suddenly, he'll go days without much contact, ghosting her. Turning off his phone for hours and becoming unreachable.

When Mia goes for a job interview for a new student job in mid-December, Ben tags along. His reasons for doing so aren't immediately clear to me. But later, Mia tells me about that afternoon, and I understand his intentions.

He's a know-it-all, wanting to be her adviser and decision-maker. Right after the interview, he tries to talk her out of the job. Mia tells me about it reluctantly. She downplays his behavior. He thinks the job is too far from her university, she says. And it's not really suited for her anyway. A call center where people call in about car breakdowns. She doesn't even have a driver's license and knows nothing about cars.

"He should mind his own business," I answer when she tells me about it. His words make me angry. He's always meddling in her affairs. "If you like the job, take it. It's solely your decision."

Your decision, your life, and your future, I add in my mind. But I wonder what role this Ben will play in your future. And what it's doing to you.

– Chapter 7 –

March 2018

"Sometimes I hate the boss when she's constantly yelling at us," Mia explains in early March.

We're sitting on a café terrace, enjoying our cappuccinos in the spring sun.

"No wonder people keep quitting and jumping ship to the competition. I won't be able to endure it much longer if she keeps this up."

"I don't get it. What's her problem?" I ask.

"Nothing satisfies her. Supposedly, we're too slow, give out the wrong information to customers, and so on and so forth. She always finds something. Yesterday, she tore the headphones off my head to end one of my client calls. I was on the verge of tears."

"Does it even make sense to keep this student job, Mia?" I ask, concerned and frustrated, at the same time. "I mean, you're supposed to stay away from stress, and now you have to deal with such a boss. You should quit and find something else," I try to convince her.

She stirs thoughtfully in her cappuccino.

"But the money is so tempting. I haven't heard of any student job that pays this well. And I'm not sure if I want to let it go," she replies.

"Mia, what good is all that money if it ends up making you sick because of someone like her? It's not worth it. If you ask me, you should quit sooner rather than later."

"You're probably right. Maybe I should apply to the rival company, like everyone else."

You should do that, I think at this moment. Because since

the beginning of the year, she's been racing through her jam-packed schedule.

She gets up at six in the morning, races to catch the bus to university. In the early afternoon, she tries to catch the bus from the university to work after her lectures, to ensure she arrives there on time.

Some of the students at work don't take punctuality seriously, she explains to me. But the arrival time can't be concealed by the company entrance card, and the boss's reaction is bound to happen.

She says she doesn't need that. The yelling as soon as you step into the office. So, she prefers to be on time.

Occasionally, she asks the lecturers at university if she can leave a lecture early. Otherwise, she won't make it to work.

Some are understanding. Others don't care about the obligations students have after university.

For Mia, that means she's sitting on pins and needles in the lecture for the last few minutes. Because she knows what awaits her at the office forty-five minutes later if she's late.

This job obviously isn't good for her, I think for the umpteenth time since she started there.

Initially, everything seemed promising. She liked the work atmosphere, the colleagues were nice, and there was no reason to complain about the boss.

Today, two months later, it's a different story, and I worry how long this can go on.

After all, stress is one of the main factors that could trigger a new relapse. Especially now, she can't afford to deal with that. Not when her relationship with Ben is already taking such a toll on her. This constant up and down.

Often, I wonder how that might affect her health. Especially when she's finally feeling as good as she has in a long time. So why all these unnecessary problems with work and Ben? Things that could be sorted out.

She could quit the job. However, it seems she's having a hard time letting go of this Ben on the other hand.

June 2018

For some inexplicable reason, since the diagnosis two years ago, we've never considered that Mia might need physiotherapy. Especially not during the times when she was doing well. As well as she is now, actually. Strangely, none of the doctors have ever pointed out that physiotherapy could benefit her. However, because I still occasionally research online about what to do with MS, even when her health condition is stable, an idea strikes me in early June.

We need a physiotherapist. I've read that muscles and mobility should be trained even when the patient is doing well, to maintain what works.

So, one afternoon, I call Sonya, the head of the MS support group. The physiotherapist needs to be enthusiastic, I explain to her, because Mia can't deal with sluggish people. She laughs at this small but important note and recommends Ethan to me. A very nice and highly competent physiotherapist who makes home visits.

Over the phone the next day, I explain to him that Mia is doing great, but it couldn't hurt for her to do something in that direction. And just a few days later, it's time. The first physiotherapy session is scheduled.

Ethan is a little over thirty, married, with a young daughter. And he also has MS. Mia says that reassures her. It gives her the feeling of being understood.

He's doing just as great, he explains when he introduces himself to us. Otherwise, he couldn't do his job, he jokes. He brings a physiotherapy table, which I'm only familiar with from massages. Honestly, I had envisioned him using an exercise ball and a yoga mat. But with the heavy table under his arm, he looks professional and well-prepared.

And then I sit in the living room chair to watch how everything unfolds over the next forty-five minutes. First, he asks Mia how she's doing. What she can and can't do. She says she can do everything, and the subtle pride in her gaze, visible only to me, doesn't escape my notice. I smile, feeling happy that she's in a position to respond to him like this.

Then come the exercises. Lasting a little over half an hour.

The sessions aren't cheap, I think to myself occasionally. But he's done his homework. You can practically see the exercise plan in his mind's eye.

Every now and then, I inquire about how we can do certain exercises on our own. On the days when he's not here. Because already, I've decided that Ethan will come to us regularly. He patiently demonstrates each exercise to Mia and explains exactly what it's for. And he keeps praising her, remarking on how well she's doing everything. Because no matter what exercise he shows her, she performs it as if she's never done anything else.

Quietly, I sit in the armchair and watch her. How ambitious she is. How well she can do everything and how happy it makes her.

Then comes the walking exercise. She's supposed to walk back and forth in the living room. I follow Ethan's gaze attentively, trying to see what he sees.

"Great. Just a tiny flaw in your gait on the right side," he explains.

I look at him puzzled. "Well, I can't see anything there. Where do you see that?"

"Mia, could you walk slowly over to the door one more time?" he asks her.

"You see, there's a tiny hitch in her knee on the right side," he points out.

As I still look at him with a question, he smiles and explains, "Maybe only I, as a physiotherapist, can see that. But that doesn't mean much."

Well, I think. He sees something I don't. No more, no less. Mia is doing great. That's all that matters.

In the following weeks, the situation with Ben escalates. Mia eagerly anticipates their meetings amidst her university and work commitments. Yet, he repeatedly disregards her obvious affection with indifference and condescension. She almost seems to be dependent on him. When I confront her about it, she defends him and makes excuses. Why does she put up with it, I ask her. But she simply responds that she doesn't see it that way.

And once again, I'm left with no choice but to concede. Because as her mother, there's not much I can do. Nothing… except for constantly trying to make her see his behavior.

Often, she sits in the bathroom late at night, crying. Of course, she doesn't want me to hear, so she flushes the toilet repeatedly when she blows her nose. When I knock and ask if everything's okay, she just replies, "Yes, I'll be out in a minute."

In those moments, I remember being young once too. She doesn't want to be alone. She wants to feel safe and understood. Unfortunately, she's chosen the wrong person for that.

What's worse is that she knows it. She knows he's wrong for her. And she knows his controlling behavior is intentional, to make her dependent and to feel superior.

What does that jerk gain from taking out his moods and low self-esteem on my daughter? I get worked up every time Tony and I discuss Mia's relationship with Ben. "I just don't know how to get her away from him anymore," I say.

"You know how it is," he tries to reassure me. "You're just her mother. She has to see it for herself. All you can do is keep talking to her about it."

And Tony is right. Because after some time, it has come to the point where Mia complains to me about Ben's behavior.

For instance, she sends him text messages that he apparently doesn't even read. On days when they have plans. Days when she's at home waiting for his signal to get ready. A text message saying he's almost ready and they can meet up.

Then, when he finally responds hours later, she asks him, "Didn't you get my text? We had plans."

And he'd say, "Yeah, I saw the text, just hadn't opened it yet. Didn't think it was urgent."

His usual condescending tone would be evident in his voice. The quiet triumph. Mia explains to me that he's one of those people who always wants to be in control. She just doesn't understand why he's doing this to her. The nicer she is to him, the more distant he becomes. Most of the time, she feels like he actually enjoys these situations. He's making her sick and doesn't seem to care.

Through tears, she admits she doesn't recognize herself anymore. She's no longer the Mia who doesn't tolerate things. The one who calls the shots.

She's afraid of being alone and tolerates his behavior because of it. Even though she knows it's not good for her. But who would want her with a disease like MS anyway, she says.

Additionally, Mia wants to quit her job but keeps getting sucked back into signing up for the new duty roster. She says she's gotten used to it. Used to the work, the colleagues, the customer calls, and the feeling of accomplishment. Yet, she sent out an application to a rival company last weekend, where many former colleagues from her current job have moved.

"Let's see. If they take me, maybe I'll quit here. Actually, the boss isn't around that much. It's not usually so bad," she says.

But I see it as excuses. She needs to quit this job for good. Just like she needs to finally get rid of Ben.

Then, one Friday at the end of June, I suddenly notice Mia's right leg occasionally buckling. A few days ago, she finally finished her university exams.

When I bring up her leg, she responds reservedly. She thinks it's from sitting too long at university and work, she replies. Some days it's up to thirteen hours.

I'm unsure and don't know what to make of it. Should I call Doctor Harper right away? Or should I wait and see if the weakness in her leg subsides on its own?

When she starts dragging her leg just a few days later, I feel a wave of panic rising within me. The fear of what might be coming next paralyzes every thought I have. Again.

Tony drives her to the university and then to work for a week. In the evenings, he picks her up by car. She explains that she doesn't want to quit this job until she has another one lined up. It will pass, she says, and she seems to genuinely believe it.

However, at the end of the week, she refuses to sign up for the new work schedule. Within just a few days, walking becomes increasingly difficult for her. I can see her disappointment as she realizes she needs to take a break because she can't go on like that.

So, she stays home. Not attending lectures or leaving the house for any reason. Some days, I have to accompany her to the bathroom to ensure she makes it on time. In her current condition she can't be around people, she explains. She doesn't even want to see Ben. Because there's certainly no support to be expected from him.

But despite all this, she still wants the new job. She insists that her walking issues will pass, as she's already received an invitation to an interview from the rival company.

"How do you envision this, Mia?" I ask her. "Just look at how you're feeling. How are you supposed to go to a job interview like this?"

"I don't know," she answers, and her expression tells me how she must be feeling. "But the email said that you could also have a first interview over the phone."

On one hand, I'm aware of the situation and only think about when it's time to call Doctor Harper. On the other hand, I want to help her. I don't want to crush her hope for a new job. Even though the prospect of this future job might be deceiving us. Making us believe that everything is okay. That these setbacks are only temporary and we don't have to worry.

"Then let's do it. Prepare for the interview and get it over with. After all, no one can see how you're feeling over the phone. Then you can still go for an in-person interview at the company once you've recovered."

"The problem is just the bathroom," she explains, looking at me questioningly. "How am I supposed to manage that if I constantly feel the urge to urinate? I can't exactly get up and go to the bathroom during the interview."

"Well, you're right. What do you suggest?" I ask, and we look at each other.

Without needing to say it out loud, the answer is written all over our faces. We need a diaper.

The preparation for the job interview a week later seems so absurd that Mia and I burst into tears of laughter. She sits on the couch dressed in diapers and a T-shirt, and we try to go over potential questions. But her responses keep making us burst into laughter.

"What are you doing besides university at the moment?"

"Well, most of the time I'm sitting at home on the couch in diapers, getting waited on."

"What about your availability for work? What hours could you work?"

"Well, actually none. I can neither stand nor sit for long. And walking is out of the question. It's best if we keep the working hours pretty short."

"And when could you start?"

"As soon as I get the next dose of corticosteroids. Then I can really hit the ground running again."

"Okay, then we have one last question. Where do you see yourself in five years?" I ask her, laughing and mimicking her fictional phone interviewer.

But as the possible answer to this simple question suddenly dawns on both of us, we fall silent and just look at each other.

What will her life be like in five years, I wonder, and I can see that she's thinking the same thing. What will she still be able to do, or not do, by then? How advanced will the disease be by then?

All these questions. They scare me, momentarily paralyzing me.

Apparently, Mia made a good impression at the rival company. During the interview, they even hinted at scheduling a face-to-face meeting at their office.

She's visibly pleased with the outcome of her conversation with the HR manager. But she can't make a personal appearance in her current state. Even if Tony were to drive her and accompany her inside, she couldn't sit there for more than ten minutes without needing the restroom constantly.

Plus, she doesn't want her limp to spoil the first impression, she explains.

So she deftly puts off the HR manager, saying she works late after classes. That's why she can only come for a personal interview in a week or two.

The HR manager assures her they're definitely interested in her joining the team, and for now, we're relieved.

Let's just wait for the flare-up to pass, I think to myself as Mia tells me about it. Then she can quit her current job and confidently accept the new one.

I almost feel a sense of anticipation over this glimmer of hope in Mia's daily life.

But there's one more thing that's been weighing on my mind. For days, I've been contemplating how to handle our holiday guests on the island this year. Currently, it's unclear what will happen with Mia's leg and her treatment. That's why I've been declining new booking requests.

However, several bookings have already been made, and we'll need to start preparing the house in the coming days to ensure it's ready on time. After all, it's already the end of June.

Our first guests would have usually arrived by now, and the thought of it alone is overwhelming.

My mother doesn't want to handle the guests alone either. She's worried about Mia, and it's all too much for her.

So, after much deliberation, I decide to simply cancel the existing bookings. Well, I think one afternoon, what needs to be done, needs to be done.

But what do you say to the guests in such a situation, I wonder as I later stare at the booking portal interface.

Sorry, no well-deserved vacation with us this year. Or maybe: Come back next year, we're taking an unplanned break this year.

Ultimately, I opt for the truth. Even though it's difficult for me. Because, in reality, this topic isn't meant for our holiday guests. After all, they've booked a vacation with sun, sea, and lots of happiness. Mind you! Without MS or related issues.

What do I do if someone doesn't understand the situation and leaves me a bad review online? Intentionally ruining my painstakingly earned reviews. Reviews that don't just reflect a stay I casually prepared in our vacation rental. But rather, they represent guests' inquiries, meticulously addressed via email for months leading up to their arrival. The organization of arrival and departure. Pick up here, drop off there. Day trips, wine tastings, kayaking, and other wishes that I accommodate during their stay. Always ready for a friendly chat, a smile, a restaurant recommendation, another towel, a thicker pillow, or even an additional fan despite air conditioning. Can you do this, can you do that, no matter what it is.

And then, is one single review supposed to ruin all of that?

July 2018

"Tomorrow, Ben and I are going to the public viewing," Mia explains in the first week of July.

The football World Cup is on, and usually Tony, Mia, and I watch the exciting games together on TV. With the obligatory bag of chips, drinks, and snacks. Now that Mia is constantly at home, we're trying to pass the time together until her recovery as best as we can.

It's only been a few days since Mia received corticosteroid infusions at the Neurology Clinic again. It was unavoidable, Doctor Harper said. Apparently, a relapse had been brewing for some time and needed to be treated as soon as possible.

Unlike usual, Mia's excitement about meeting Ben this time seems rather subdued—and that surprises me. Surely it's been more than two weeks since they last saw each other.

When I ask if he had even reached out during that time, she explains that he had actually been nicer than usual.

On one hand, I'm glad to hear that. Nevertheless, I don't like the idea of her meeting him. Because I'm still skeptical, and I can't quite trust this sudden change.

"Great. At least you'll get out of the house," I reply, not wanting to dampen her spirits.

In truth, I find him dreadful and would prefer to do something to keep her away from him. Persuade her not to see him, to protect her from him in a way.

But it's not my place to interfere, I remind myself again.

The next day, Mia leaves the house around three in the afternoon. It's oppressively hot outside, and she should really be staying away from the sun right now. But she's determined to meet Ben.

Tony has hastily procured crutches for her from the pharmacy. Until now, she wanted nothing to do with them. But now she can't manage without a mobility aid, and she's aware of it. Apparently, this meeting is worth the embarrassment she must feel. After all, just a few days ago, she adamantly stated that she wouldn't be caught dead in public with crutches.

Nevertheless, she seems relieved as I bid her farewell at the door.

I wait a few minutes until she's walked down the stairs and onto the street. Then I stand at the window and watch her from behind closed curtains.

I almost feel ashamed, and my stomach knots up as I watch her walk down the street like that.

Her sight is almost unbearable for a moment.

What has happened to her carefree life? Where has it gone? For a moment, I'm overwhelmed by a feeling I've never known before. The indescribable fear of life. Fear of a life that seems to be out of my control. A life that determines itself how it goes on and what the next day will bring. I'm no longer the director. Someone else has long taken over the pen and continues writing the lines of our lives arbitrarily.

And that scares me.

"It's over. I broke up with him," Mia explains, visibly upset, as she comes home later that evening.

Her mascara is smudged. Obviously, she cried on the way home.

"Where does he get the right to treat me like that? He can screw off. I'm not putting up with this anymore," she continues in one breath, unable to calm down.

As I help her take off her shoes in the hallway, she breaks into tears again.

"What happened, Mia?" I ask, concerned about how she got home. Maybe he left her alone at the café. "Come, sit down for a moment. Then you can tell me what's going on."

"There's nothing to tell. Ben's an idiot," she explains, sobbing. "Do you know what he asked me yesterday when we were supposed to meet? If I still limp? Can you imagine? Like, what's he gonna do with someone like me? And when I got to the corner today, he just looked at me stupidly. I could tell he was ashamed of me."

"What's going on?" Tony calls from the living room. He's probably wondering about our loud conversation in the hallway.

"Nothing. We just need to talk about something," I call back. He must hear in my tone that I want to sort something out alone with Mia.

Shortly after, we're in her room. She's lowered the blinds on the windows and sits at her vanity.

"Do you want to talk about it, Mia?" I try to start the conversation.

Tears still stream down her cheeks as she removes her makeup.

And suddenly, there's that familiar silence from her.

She actually doesn't want to talk about it, I realize. He must have hurt her so deeply that she can't bring herself to speak of it. Not now. Maybe later, when she's ready.

She'll give me another reason for the unexpected breakup with Ben. Just moments ago at the door, she seemed willing to say something. But now, within just a few minutes, she retreats. She'll keep it to herself, so I won't learn the true reason for their rift.

There have been too many of these situations lately, and I know I won't hear the actual events of this afternoon for now.

"Maybe you'll feel better if you talk about it," I try again.

"There's nothing to tell. We were sitting there. He was eyeing other women the whole time and telling me about a summer job he applied for. That's it for me. I'm too good for that," she says.

That can't be all, I think again. However, I keep my thoughts to myself.

"But that's not why you broke up," I reply, waiting for her reaction.

"He seriously asked me if I wanted to come along. There were other summer jobs available," she explains. "How am I supposed to go anywhere like this?" she continues, pointing to her legs. "It's ridiculous. He knows perfectly well I can't go."

"Okay, and what did you say to that?"

"First of all that it's not possible, and secondly, it's not even a job for me. Then he just shrugged. As if he couldn't care less. He asked, I said no. And that was the end of the conversation. So we won't see each other all summer."

"And that's it?" I ask, surprised.

She hesitates for a moment, and I can tell she wants to say something. But she only nods and then goes to the bathroom to wash her face, as she says.

And to quietly cry about what you can't tell me right now, I add silently.

– Chapter 8 –

Friday in August 2018

This summer, every day in the city feels stiflingly hot. The first weeks of August pass by, and Mia's health condition worsens noticeably.

Once again, it starts with the right side of her body. She can't even put weight on her already weakened right leg anymore. Additionally, her right arm is now hardly usable, she says.

But this time, her right eye is also affected. As if all of that wasn't enough. She describes it as seeing through a broken television. When watching TV, she wears her reading glasses with a tissue over the right lens so she doesn't have to look through that eye constantly.

I keep thinking about how much has changed in such a short time when I look at her. It's been less than a month since the corticosteroids, and another treatment would be too soon. However, she can't stay like this. She can neither walk properly nor do anything else independently.

During the day, Mia and I limp together to the bathroom; she eats and brushes her teeth using only her left hand. In the evenings, she's so exhausted that Tony has to carry her to bed.

Right now, I should stay away from internet information. But I can't help it. In the evenings, while Mia sleeps, I read about breathing difficulties and swallowing problems. About the lasting damages relapses can cause if not stopped in time. The thought of all that can happen drives me crazy.

That's why throughout the day, I find myself repeatedly picking up my phone, almost calling Doctor Harper. But Mia wants to wait until it gets better. On its own. She doesn't want to poison her body with those infusions again, she explains in those moments.

However, I'm increasingly doubtful that it will actually get better with each passing day, and this sudden progression of the disease scares me.

On a Friday morning at the end of August, the moment comes when I can't bear to see Mia's condition any longer. Her condition is deteriorating by the hour, and I don't care how long it has been since her last treatment. In past conversations, they reassured us that she has received the best medication available and there is nothing else. But I don't care about that now. They have to do something, no matter what, as long as it's quick. Who knows how long it will take for all these deficits to revert to normal. I shudder at the thought of any lingering effects—dragging her leg, limping, a weakened hand, or an eye that can't see properly.

The panic sets in just thinking about it. Because the longer the symptoms persist, the more difficult the recovery will surely be, I tell myself. It just has to go away. Right away.

So, at eight in the morning, I quickly pack a few things into a small overnight bag. Her pajamas, toothbrush, some toiletries, and her phone charger. I remember the packing list from her last hospital stay. Mia mentions that it wouldn't hurt to bring a diaper for the trip just before Tony carries her to the car.

Then it's off to the emergency room.

When we arrive at around five in the evening, the neurology department's hallway is bustling with activity. A male nurse wheels Mia's bed to a patient room and asks us to wait just outside until another nurse arrives.

Apparently, they're preparing the evening meal for the patients. A food trolley stands in the middle of the hallway, and the air is filled with the scent of potato soup and eggs.

Earlier, after a long wait in the emergency room, a doctor had told us that Mia needed to be admitted urgently. "We consulted with Doctor Harper. Today's his day off. However, he believes it's best to admit her to Neurology Ward 6 for now. We'll conduct a few tests first," she added.

At some point around noon, I found myself wondering when these examinations would finally come to an end. When a nurse once again attempted to measure Mia's blood pressure, I brought up the long wait we endured in the emergency room.

"Sorry, we don't have a bed available in neurology right now. We'll have to wait until the afternoon until something is arranged," she briefly explained before disappearing again.

Now that we're finally on the neurology ward, I'm annoyed to find ourselves waiting once more. From the snippets of conversation among the nurses, I gather they're trying to find a suitable room for Mia.

Perhaps one without elderly patients in the throes of illness. Memories of the last stay linger unpleasantly in my mind. It wasn't pleasant. Especially not for a twenty-four-year-old in this situation.

Shortly after, a spot in Room 9 becomes available. The head nurse instructs us to wait outside for a moment while Mia's diaper is changed in the patient's room. Just as one of the nurses is about to wheel Mia's bed into the prepared room, Mia reaches for my hand.

"Mom," she whispers, and I lean in close to her. "I don't want this," she explains, tears of desperation streaming down her cheeks. "I'm twenty-four. Can you please do the diaper?" The pleading in her eyes tugs at my heartstrings.

"Of course, sweetie, I'll just sort it out with the nurses," I reply, kissing her forehead.

Until now, it's only been her and I who could laugh off this diaper situation at home. Now, there are hospital nurses who merely carry out their daily tasks, ignoring the patients' embarrassment. Where could their understanding possibly lead, I wonder. Embarrassment, compassion, accommodation. All of it is time-consuming and therefore out of place in their daily routine.

"I'm sorry. That's the nurses' job," the head nurse responds sharply to my request. "You won't be here in the next few days, so we'll handle it."

"But at least for now, I could take care of it. Mia's had a long day," the pleading in my voice is unmistakable, but her response is evident even before she speaks.

"Unfortunately, I can't let you into the patient's room. And you certainly won't change the diaper in the hallway."

She didn't say that, I think angrily. I meet her eyes, wanting to vent my frustration, to complain, to yell at her. But in the next moment, I realize that arguing in this situation would be futile. Despite my anger, I must keep my composure. After all, my child will be at the mercy of these nurses' goodwill in the coming days. Whether I like it or not.

So, Tony and I remain outside the room while Mia, in tears, has her diaper changed inside.

Meanwhile, I silently weep by the door.

Finally, the workweek at the hospital has started again, I think on Monday morning. Two days have passed since Mia's admission last Friday, and they immediately started administering corticosteroids to her on the same evening. It turns out, as I thought. Even though the last therapy wasn't that long ago. Nobody talks about it, but I have the feeling that they're not quite sure what else to give her.

Last Friday in the emergency room, they said Doctor Harper had a day off. Now, however, Mia told me he's on vacation, and a Doctor Winters is covering for him in the meantime.

Yesterday, I visited her for the first time in her office on the Neurology Ward, and I found her immediately off-putting. When I asked what treatment plan she discussed with Doctor Harper, she responded snippily and shortly. I wanted to know what the next steps were. But she didn't even look at me while I stood beside her. She stared blankly at some documents on her desk.

Freshly dyed blonde highlights in her hair, seemingly attempting to conceal the inevitable gray. A neatly drawn eyeliner and, in my opinion, a lipstick shade a bit too bright.

Apparently, the daily competition among colleagues doesn't suit her, I thought in that moment. Which doctor is more competent, more experienced, and who can still hope for a promotion? And of course, the tiresome topic: who is prettier? Who can still attract the attention of the still dominant male colleagues in this work environment. After all, amidst everything else, she is still a woman.

"Doctor Winters. The person in Room 9 is my daughter, and I want to know what Mia will be administered in the coming days. If you can't provide an answer, I'll gladly call Doctor Harper myself. I have no issue with that."

Suddenly, she looked up, narrowing her eyes at me. Then she leaned back in her office chair.

"That won't be necessary," was her response to my provocation, and I could practically see her boiling with anger.

"Okay, then we have that settled. So, what's the plan moving forward?"

On Tuesday evening around 7 p.m., Tony and I are in the car on our way home. We've just come from the hospital. Mia seemed cheerful. As always, I think. But I can't smile about it.

Instead, I stare out the passenger window. I only vaguely register the passing streets, houses, and people. Why aren't these damn corticosteroids helping her anymore, I wonder, fighting back tears. We've always been able to rely on their quick action before. One or two infusions, and we could always see some small progress. A glimmer of hope that it would soon be over.

But this time it's different. Mia is getting weaker day by day. Both legs are affected now. She can't even move a toe anymore. Paralyzed, immobile, with no feeling in her limbs.

Her right arm is numb now. Lifting it properly or moving her fingers is impossible. What was manageable last night during our hospital visit is impossible today. Incapable of movement. Every sensation and every trace of life in her arms and legs is fading away like clockwork. As if the nerve pathways are wearily closing their eyes and drifting into a deep sleep. Into an endless anesthesia. Deeper and deeper. Silent and motionless.

Her sight is difficult for me to bear. She lies there in her hospital bed. The side rails raised to prevent her from falling out. Day in and day out. Clad only in a diaper and a tank top. In temperatures over ninety degrees in the stuffy room, without even a hint of a breeze. Helpless and at the mercy of the everyday, repetitive rituals of hospital life.

At six sharp every morning, a nurse comes to her bedside. With a basin and disposable washcloths.

"Would you like the yellow or the purple shower gel today, Mia?" she asks, smiling.

"Purple is fine," Mia replies.

She pours some of the shower gel into the basin and dips the disposable washcloth into the warm water. Then she starts washing Mia. Methodically, from head to toe. Always smiling.

At least, that's how it is when the nice nurse is on duty. She talks to her at least, Mia later recounts. It's not exactly great being bathed by someone as an adult. Conversation is a good distraction. When you're being maneuvered around in bed like a sack of potatoes because you can't move your own body anymore.

Unfortunately, there are also nurses who don't place much value on human connection with the patient. Not a word is spoken. The tasks are simply carried out. "There, you're all set. Next!" they seem to say, eager to move on quickly.

"Breakfast is coming soon," is all they offer, and then the nurse leaves the room as if Mia were just a piece of furniture she had wiped down.

Fortunately, she has her two roommates, I often think. They're nice. Older ladies. One is here because of a minor stroke, the other due to unexplained behavioral changes. They say they don't mind being here. They've already lived their lives. But what about Mia? This young life. Just getting started. I remain silent when they say this. What can I even say in response.

They have their routines, Mia tells me during visiting hours. They watch the news together. After dinner, Maria always peels an orange for them. Then they pray and sing. And afterward, they watch old TV shows. It's not necessarily Mia's first choice, but you make do in this monotonous hospital routine.

A routine where meals, morning rounds, and afternoon visits from family and friends are the highlights of the day. Mia says they eagerly anticipate these moments, constantly staring at the door. Hoping someone brings a small piece of the outside world into the microcosm of the hospital room. From a world where everything is still intact. Completely normal. Unlike here in the hospital. Where the oppressive sounds from other rooms echo down the hallway. Moans, cries, weeping, the incessant calls for the nurses.

Add to that the smells. Full urine bags, vomit, and sweat. And that indescribable odor of age and illness. Because most here are indeed old. Every day she must endure that. Trapped in her own body, as she puts it. Unable to escape it. Simply getting up and leaving.

All that would be over quickly, I think now as we drive. Her sufferings, this uncertainty. Everything. If only the treatment with the corticosteroids would work. Whereas the promising wonder drug has already failed.

But they just don't help anymore. And what Mia just revealed to me is another shock. During the morning rounds, she was informed that tomorrow she would undergo something called plasmapheresis. Because the corticosteroids are no longer effective.

Plasma… what? That must be something to do with blood, I thought at that moment. They said it's like blood washing, she explained when I asked further.

Blood washing. But what exactly?

"Didn't they explain how it works? And more importantly, why you need it."

"No, they didn't. They always rush through their rounds. Quick glance, whispered consultation, and off they go. There's no time for questions. I mean, I'd like to know what they're doing to me."

"Well, I'll ask now," I replied.

So I went to the nurses' station to find the head nurse. Yes, a plasma exchange was deemed necessary by the neurologists, she replied. And it starts tomorrow morning. Why nobody informed me about this. After all, it's obviously not a minor issue.

She avoided my gaze. "The doctors decided that, and Mia was notified during the morning rounds," she said.

That was supposed to mean: That's enough. Why should anyone explain it to you.

It seems they couldn't care less that Mia is hardly receptive anymore due to all the infusions, painkillers, and sleeping pills, I thought, irritated by such ignorance. Mia doesn't even know what was served for breakfast. Whether she was washed by the nurses today or yesterday. Let alone does she have the strength to inquire exactly how this plasma thing is supposed to work.

"And what's the plasma exchange for? I mean, why is it being done? Is it routine or should I be worried?"

"I can't say. That's Doctor Harper's decision. You'd better ask the doctors tomorrow," the head nurse replied.

Short and to the point. And not very helpful either.

"But didn't you just say it's happening tomorrow morning? When am I supposed to ask then? If I'm not mistaken, visiting hours are only in the afternoon." This head nurse is really starting to annoy me, I thought, squinting at her.

"Well, then ask in the afternoon." And she had that triumphant look again. Patronizing.

"If everything's already happening. Great," I replied.

Apparently, nobody thinks it's necessary to inform us about the details. Then I'll just google it, I thought. Like everything else. I probably can't intervene anyway. I don't know if it's good or bad, or what to make of it. A decision for or against this treatment or even a say, seems irrelevant.

Just as I was about to leave the nurses' station, the head nurse had something else to add.

"Here." She vaguely pointed with her right index finger to the area below her collarbone. "Here, they make an incision. Over there, they insert the access. That's all I can say."

Wednesday, first day of plasmapheresis

The next morning, around nine, I'm at the computer, busy translating. Since I woke up, I've had this uneasy feeling in my stomach about the plasmapheresis. Then, I get a text from Mia.

"All good, alive," it says, followed by a smiling emoji.

Those three words ease my mind a bit after last night. The uncertainty about when they'll insert the access and start the blood washing kept me up. I tossed and turned in bed all night. My internet research didn't exactly help me calm down.

Of course, I spent last night delving into it further. But it didn't ease my mind.

The descriptions. Proteins are separated from the plasma. The photos, the tubes. On the arm, collarbone, or neck. Fortunately, the head nurse mentioned the collarbone. That's manageable, I thought as I looked at the photos.

But as I open the attachment to Mia's seemingly cheerful text message on this Wednesday morning, it leaves me breathless.

She lies in her hospital bed. Only her upper body and head are visible. A light blue sheet covers her obviously unclothed upper body. Shoulders and arms exposed.

As if my mind filters the information in the photo, my gaze initially focuses only on the bed. The headrest is slightly raised and covered with a dark green sheet.

Like after surgery, it occurs to me. Her long golden-brown hair is completely covered with a cap. She keeps her eyes half-closed. I try to interpret her expression. Neutral, I would say. Yes, neutral. As if she's thinking, "Well, at least I've got it over with now." Just as I know her.

And then I allow it. My gaze shifts to what this photo is meant to show.

To the right, just a few centimeters from her larynx, protrudes a transparent tube. From a fresh incision in her neck.

So, it is, I think, and my stomach clenches. So, it really is her neck.

By now, it's nearly four in the afternoon. Tony and I are standing outside the glass door of the Neurology Ward. Visiting hours are about to begin, and a nurse opens the door for us as she spots us.

Today, I've brought Mia's favorite meal: lentil stew. Packed in a Tupperware and wrapped in foil to keep it warm. Actually, it wouldn't be necessary in this summer heat, but I've wrapped everything meticulously. Today, of all days, I want to bring her a little piece of home to the hospital. Especially after experiencing that plasma procedure for the first time this morning, along with the early intervention.

The neurology ward seems busier than usual today, I think, spotting Doctor Winters outside Room 9, talking loudly on the phone and pacing anxiously. Two nurses rush in and out of the room.

"What's going on here?" I ask Tony. "This is Mia's room," I add hesitantly.

And suddenly, I feel my heart racing. "Mia's room," I repeat quietly.

Hastily, I hand Tony the bag with the Tupperware and walk past Doctor Winters into Room 9.

Mia's roommate, Maria, rushes toward me with tears streaming down her face. She can barely compose herself.

"I don't know how this could happen. She was fine just a moment ago. Cheerful as ever. We were talking, and suddenly… suddenly she stopped responding. Just turned her head to the side. I went to her, but she didn't react. Then I ran out into the hallway and called for the nurse. How could this happen?"

Meanwhile, my gaze remains fixed on one thing: my child. How she lies there, with an oxygen tube in her nose and another protruding from her throat. Quiet and motionless.

I approach her bedside. "I'm here, sweetie," I whisper into her ear, gently stroking her head. She looks at me and smiles. Before she can respond, Doctor Winters suddenly appears beside me.

"Listen, that was a minor episode of weakness. I can't explain it either," her words cascade onto me. There's a hint of guilt in her tone that is impossible to miss. "But she's feeling better now," she adds quickly. "She's already opening her eyes. Mia, just nod for your mother to see that you're doing better."

"What do you mean you can't explain it?" I ask louder than intended, locking eyes with her. "Didn't you check if Mia was even suitable for this plasma treatment beforehand? I mean, is her body even strong enough for something like this right now?"

"Well, given the circumstances, there wasn't much to assess. We had to act. And plasma exchange is a proven method in her situation," she responds.

In her situation … I repeat in my mind. I'm well aware of what her situation looks like. And it scares me.

"We can't do anything else for her," she adds, and for the first time, I see something akin to pity in her gaze.

They're at a loss, I realize. The doctors at a loss. They have no more tricks up their sleeves. No miracle cure. Just this plasma thing. A final effort before the end. It'll probably be said then:

She's reached the end of available treatments. Like in tragic TV dramas. We can't do anything more. Paralyzed and entirely dependent on others for help.

Quickly, I push away that thought.

"Will the treatment be continued?" I ask. "And what interests me most, what does Doctor Harper say about this? Does he know what's going on?"

My own words ignite a sense of determination within me. They won't get rid of us that easily, I think in the next moment. There's always something we can do.

"Of course. I just informed him about Mia's condition over the phone. And yes, we will continue the treatment," she explains.

"Well then, it's about time you explain to me exactly what this is all about and how long it's going to take," I reply.

Tony is meanwhile sitting on a chair beside Mia's bed, holding her hand. He looks at me, as if to say, "Calm down."

I wish I could just settle this with the doctor in the hallway, I think to myself. But he's right. Mia doesn't need this commotion right now. On top of everything else she's gone through today. I want to be with her, to keep an eye on her while I talk to the doctor.

"So, how long will this blood treatment take?" I ask, more calmly.

"The first session was this morning, and there will be four more to follow. Alternating with the corticosteroids. One day plasmapheresis, the next corticosteroids. For a total of ten days," she explains.

"Thank you," I reply, sinking onto the edge of Mia's bed. Suddenly, I feel unbelievably tired. I just want this doctor to leave the room. I want her to close the door and to take her thoughts and words with her. So I can, for a brief moment, make my daughter's world right again in this small patient room. With my lentil stew. With our stories from home. With Tony's jokes. With Mia's smile.

Thursday

The next day, around ten in the morning, Mia sends me a text message. Just as I finish my first translation task of the day. She wants me to call her.

"Doctor Harper is back," she tells me.

Then she recounts in detail the morning visit, amused once again by her neurologist's restrained demeanor. He had come to her room shortly after breakfast, unexpectedly. A glance at the chart at the foot of her bed, and he was by her side, inquiring about her well-being. "Well, could be better," she replied. Suddenly, he uncovered her blanket at the foot of the bed and looked at her toes. "Move them," he instructed. But, nothing happened. She gave him a look that said, "What did you expect? Nothing works."

She shrugged with a smile. Smiling at the unspoken humor they both understood. And smiling at the absurdity of the situation. A toe was supposed to fix it all. Just a small movement and there would be a glimmer of hope. For doctor and patient.

Then, he left the room silently once again.

During our afternoon visit, if he has finally said anything about what comes next. When the therapy will finally take effect. Initially, I planned to ask him all of this myself. Now that he's finally back at work. Yet, he remains unreachable to me. For now, I'll have to settle for Mia's insights and wait for a conversation with Doctor Harper.

As on any given day, Tony and I showed up punctually at four in the hospital room. We brought provisions from home. Snacks, fruit, water bottles with sip caps. So she won't spill while drinking. I just changed her diaper, turned her in bed, washed her, and dressed her.

Meanwhile, Tony went to a nearby café. The one overlooking the big park. Where he can unwind while we go through our caregiving routine here. And our conversations. Conversations reserved just for us. Mia and me. Her mother.

"Your hair's all tangled. I think the ponytail isn't such a good idea anymore. I should braid two side braids for you," I explain, wondering how she's really feeling. Not the supposedly cheerful Mia who always lends an ear to her older roommates. But my Mia. My child.

"Yeah, good idea. I'm just lying on my back anyway. But be careful with the tube in my throat," she replies, tilting her head gently to the side so I can start braiding the first braid.

All of a sudden, memories flood over me. Memories of braiding her hair before kindergarten, using her favorite hair ties. Those with two light green transparent balls containing a flower inside. Her long, golden-brown hair, smelling of children's shampoo. And childhood. Of sand tangled in her hair after lively afternoons at the playground. Of sunshine and her joyful laughter.

I smile as I reminisce. But as quickly as the memory came, reality pulls me back in as I hear Mia's words.

"Sometimes in the morning, after waking up, I feel like I could just get up and walk away. It's like I forget for a second that I can't. And then comes the shock. The realization. I can't even describe it. It's an unspeakable shock every time," she explains to me, her words penetrating every fiber of my being.

I think I can feel what she must feel in those moments. The brief lightness. The joy and the feeling of freedom. And then the sudden certainty. The fear.

"I feel trapped in my own body, Mom. I can't even run away from myself. You can all leave. Just walk out of the hospital and continue to live normally. But not me," she whispers, her voice choked with tears.

I lean in close to her, my face near hers, as I look into her eyes.

"Mia, it won't stay like this. We'll get rid of it! I promise you," I whisper emphatically, gently stroking her face. "I'm here, and there are always possibilities, even ones we may not know about yet. Your body will recover. You're young. We'll do everything to get you back on your feet. Believe me, it won't stay like this."

Yet, what must I do to make that happen? I add silently in my thoughts.

Monday, September 3, 2017

On Monday morning, I slowly begin to grasp that Mia's recovery might take longer this time, and the doctors obviously don't know what to do. It's already September 3rd, and time appears to be slipping away from us. Until today, I refused to admit it, feeling like a runner with the finish line in sight, just needing to make that final sprint. But now, that goal seems to have vanished from my view, and I have no idea how much further the journey will be. I seem to have long since lost control over Mia's progress, feeling a sense of panic and helplessness that keeps me awake at night.

Even Mia's consistently good spirits and the kind bedmates in her hospital room, who dote on her, can't mask the true situation anymore. Mia, at twenty-four, lies paralyzed and in diapers in the neurology ward, and her condition hasn't changed since she was admitted over ten days ago.

Yesterday, Sunday, she had a visit from her academic advisor, Mrs. Angel. She didn't want to inquire about Mia's health status just over the phone or via email anymore. She wanted to see Mia to personally tell her not to worry about the last exam. Mia kept talking about this exam. She didn't want to fall behind and start the next academic year with unresolved issues. But that's not so important right now, Mrs. Angel explained to her while sitting by Mia's bedside on Sunday afternoon.

When she entered the room at her arrival, I saw her puzzled expression. Then the obvious concern at Mia's appearance, which she tried to hide. But what didn't escape me: her usually perfectly styled student, who shone with knowledge and enthusiasm in every presentation and exam, now lay in front of her in diapers and a tank top.

"Excuse my appearance," Mia joked, but Mrs. Angel just smiled and placed a box of chocolates on the nightstand.

"With alcohol. But that's our little secret," she explained, still smiling, and took a seat next to Mia's bed.

A conversation followed, during which Mia shared funny anecdotes from her hospital routine with the two older ladies. Mrs. Angel laughed but remained mostly silent. She seemed amazed at the possibility of finding joy even in this situation. Mia's obvious cheerfulness seemed to perplex her.

After about twenty minutes, she bid Mia goodbye, stroking her cheek. And I glimpsed a touch of sorrow in her expression.

Who knows what thoughts crossed her mind on the journey home. Perhaps about how things may not get better. Perhaps about how she won't see Mia as the vibrant student at the university anymore, the one who eagerly occupies the front row each morning, looking forward to the upcoming lecture.

Or maybe about how today, in this hospital room, she was confronted with the fleeting, inadequate, and fragile nature of life, which can visit us all at any moment in our brief existence.

Yesterday, on Sunday, was the third plasma exchange, and now, on Monday afternoon, as I head to the hospital, I wonder how it will all continue. Tony cranked up the air conditioning to cool down, but I roll down the passenger window to breathe. To inhale the late summer scent of the city, and evoke the feeling as if it were just a normal afternoon. No worries, no special events. Maybe an afternoon where we'd drive to the city park together and sit in a café. Where we'd sip cappuccinos and discuss the upcoming grape harvest on the island. Talk about when Tony would head to the island to help his parents with the harvest. But I can't seem to escape reality. Not even in my thoughts.

Again and again, I wonder why this plasma exchange isn't working either. The last treatment is in a few days. No one seems willing—or able—to give me answers. Shouldn't you expect specialists to know what to do? No matter how serious or complicated a patient's condition is. Who will help us if not them, I keep asking myself. There must be a way to get Mia back on her feet. My Mia, who rushes to catch the bus in the morning to make it to university on time. My ordinary Mia, who enjoys her young life. Who walks like everyone else. There must be a way to stop those inflammations in her brain. It always worked before. Why not this time?

After a half-hour drive, Tony and I finally reach the neurology department, and I spot Doctor Harper in the hallway. Finally. Finally, I can ask him all my questions, I think relieved, and I walk up to him. He's here. Within reach. Now I'll grab him, and he can't run away from me. An odd thought crosses my mind. The hallway is narrow. There's a closed glass door at the end of it. He has to pass by me if he wants to go there. I almost laugh at this absurd brainstorm as Doctor Harper suddenly stands before me.

Why isn't any of this working? I ask him. What about that medication that seemed so promising?

Based on Mia's recent blood tests, they found that the number of lymphocytes prevented the previous medication from working, he says. It couldn't attach to the right cells, he further explains. Only her and one other case in the Czech Republic have been reported so far.

Why didn't anyone tell us this? I ask, struggling to contain a rising feeling of anger. They simply didn't know, he replies, looking at me.

"What do we do now?" I whisper.

I can hardly look at him because fear of the answer paralyzes me. What if he says, "Nothing. There's nothing more to be done"?

But then it comes. The answer to all my questions. A single sentence he utters. Apparently conflicted about whether he should even tell me about this possibility of recovery. He seems subdued, somehow unsure how I'll react to it. Or perhaps he's afraid I'll cling to his words. Insist on what he's hinting at. This single ray of hope. Which seems to be the last resort before there's no treatment left.

"Most likely, she'll undergo B-cell therapy."

Hardly has he uttered this sentence when his phone rings, and he's gone again. And I stand there. Lost.

Tony has meanwhile entered Mia's hospital room. I stand indecisively in the hospital corridor. Frozen in place where Doctor Harper just spoke those words to me. "Probably" echoes in my mind. What does he mean by "probably"? What is B-cell therapy, anyway? When will she receive it? Did I miss the probable date in my agitation? A week, a month? Will she even get it? How certain can we be? And how promising is this therapy compared to the previously highly praised medication?

With all these questions, he left me standing here. And with the word "probably." A word that won't leave my mind. A single small word, containing so many ifs and buts, that I'll spend the next days and nights pondering over it. I'll reevaluate the emphasis over and over again. I'll wonder how Doctor Harper pronounced that one sentence. If I misunderstood or misheard something. How his expression looked when he said those words. Confident or rather resigned? How he emphasized each word. Whether he sounded casual or entirely certain about planning this therapy for Mia.

Probably. This one word breeds fear and doubt within me. And in the next moment, a surge of excitement. The hope for a new beginning. An unexpected treatment possibility. And for a normal life.

Tuesday, 4th day of plasmapheresis

"The treatment is almost over, and there's no progress. Do you think Doctor Harper will have to order this new medication, or do they already have it in stock at the hospital? And… whether she'll even get it?" I ask Tony on Tuesday morning as we have breakfast.

It all sounded so uncertain, I add silently, trying to swallow a piece of bread. I hardly slept last night, and headaches have been bothering me since early morning.

Tony just looks at me. He knows I'm not really asking him these questions, just pondering out loud. I gaze out the kitchen window. When I briefly close my eyes, I feel the first rays of sun on my face, and I'm ashamed of a sudden sense of well-being. How can you feel okay while she's in the hospital? The thought hits me with such unexpected guilt that it almost takes my breath away. You're sitting here comfortably in the kitchen, smelling fresh coffee and basking in the sunlight? Meanwhile, she is lying there helpless. Can't move, can't even eat alone. How can you? What kind of mother are you? Joy is not for you. Not now. Not anytime soon. Focus on her. On getting her life back on track.

And then it's back. That dull ache. A pain that has become routine for me. It accompanies me through the day. Through the night. Sometimes subdued, then pushing forward again. But it's always there. It doesn't let me sleep or think clearly. Eventually, it's invaded every cell of my body and lingers there. Uninvited. Relentless. But I defy it. In my own way. I resist it by striving daily to find something positive in my current life. Like peering through a telescope into a future I envision according to my own desires. A future where my daughter Mia is healthy. Where she walks and does all the things a twenty-four-year-old should.

From this vision, I draw the necessary strength to motivate myself day in and day out. A motivation that Mia should perceive in my eyes, in every word I utter, in my gestures, my actions, and my being during each of my visits to the hospital. Every day, again and again. So that she too is carried by a hope that encourages her to keep going.

"Do you already know anything about this B-cell therapy?" Tony abruptly interrupts my pondering. "You must have looked it up online last night."

I look at him, noticing he's already on his second cup of espresso. Not good for his stomach, I think.

"Yes, of course I did," I reply, feeling his question stirring something within me.

Alongside the indescribable pain, I feel a drive to take action. Finally, there's something to grasp onto and occupy my mind. I'll research everything about this treatment option. She has to get it. As soon as possible. After this constant uncertainty, I finally have something concrete to work towards.

"Well, he didn't mention a name, but I found a medication that corresponds to this B-cell therapy. That must be what he meant. Pretty expensive. Hopefully, the insurance won't cause any problems. From what I understand, it targets the B-cells because there are too many in MS patients. An excess of these cells apparently causes inflammation." I finish my coffee, and suddenly, the uplifting feeling I had vanishes. Somewhere within me, the constant doubt lurks, preventing me from believing in the effectiveness of even the most promising medication with an unbiased mind.

"In any case, the therapy sounds good," I conclude my explanation and wonder what ›good‹ actually means. Does "good" mean it works? Or is it just another chance with an uncertain outcome?

"I mean, they made a big deal out of the last medication. Like she'd get it, and then she'd have a few years of peace. All modern," I continue my thoughts. "I don't really trust these therapies anymore," I explain with a choked voice. "But what else can we do? We don't have any other choice. She ... can't stay like this."

Actually, I rarely cry these days. Tears haven't been able to relieve me of all this pressure for a long time. However, I can't always hold them back, and it feels good to let them flow freely for a brief moment. Sitting at the kitchen table and just crying. A weeping that turns into helpless sobbing as Tony holds me in his arms. I cry tears of devastation over a fate I didn't see coming. About how the future of my child's life will apparently depend on the goodwill of others. Whether this life will even be worth living.

And I cry over the realization that every day could be crucial. That another day where her brain sends no signals to her body, where her nerves no longer function, and her limbs lie dormant, could lead to it staying that way in the future. For the rest of her life.

In the early afternoon, Tony and I attend to our daily duties. He with blueprints for his company, me with my translations. This monotonous yet reassuring routine helps me get through the day. While doing my translation tasks, I constantly drift off and can't focus on what's in front of me on the laptop screen. Not even cleaning the apartment relaxes me like it used to.

In recent weeks, it's become a manic habit to take a cold shower for minutes after visiting the hospital in the evening, then clean the apartment, only to shower again. No matter what I do, the same thoughts circle in my head. Relentlessly, the worry about Mia's future plagues me. And now the question about this new medication has come up as well. Another topic to ponder for hours until my head feels like it's going to explode.

Around two in the afternoon, I packed Mia's lunch in Tupperware containers: breaded chicken fillet and potatoes with parsley. She likes that, and it's a welcome change from the hospital meals. This morning, I searched for a smoothie recipe on the internet, one that would help with constipation. Mia's been complaining about it for days. It must be all the medications,

I told her two days ago. Today morning, a nurse informed her they wanted to wait a bit longer before giving her a laxative.

"How much longer do I have to endure this?" she asked half an hour ago on the phone.

"Not long, I'll take care of it," I reassured her.

Now I'm in the kitchen, preparing her a smoothie: with beetroot, two chopped almonds, almond milk, frozen spinach, a handful of frozen berries, freshly squeezed orange juice, a teaspoon of flaxseed, and a small piece of banana. And they said something about turmeric powder and fresh ginger on the internet. They're supposed to be anti-inflammatory, so those go in too. Well, she'll recognize the beetroot immediately by the color and probably won't be thrilled. But that's okay. Hopefully, the banana flavor will prevail. Anyway, the smoothie smells extremely enticing. I won't taste the concoction myself, though. If it really works, that wouldn't be ideal during visiting hours for me. I smile at the thought.

Then I remember her pained expression when she talks about constipation, and the smile fades. She shouldn't have to suffer from that on top of everything else, I think, as I pour the mix into a coffee cup with a lid.

But it's not just any coffee cup; it's THE coffee cup: adorned with a typical red London bus, the silhouette of the city's main landmarks, and well-dressed ladies apparently about to embark on a shopping spree. And then there's that inscription: *Bakery Bus*. We received this cup as a gift during our Bakery Bus tour of London, and now I deliberately bring it out to remind Mia of happier times. To inject a bit of optimism into her gray hospital days, hinting at another journey to London.

Meanwhile, I ask myself how she really feels. Outwardly, she appears composed and even cheerful. But what lies beneath the surface? What thoughts torment her when she lies awake at night, while her roommates sleep soundly. Alone in the darkness, with only her thoughts and the soft breathing in the room. I imagine the longing for life outside that must consume her in these nights. How vulnerable she must feel. And what future she envisions for her young life. Now, she must suddenly become a different person. Someone who can't get up, wash, dress, and prepare for the day independently.

She's no longer the Mia who grabs her purse and the blue backpack, spritzes herself with perfume in the hallway, and heads out of the house. To start a day full of vigor with morning lectures at the university and evenings that never seem to end after work. Because there's still enough youthful energy in her, and she doesn't want the day to end.

How must it feel for her to realize that this Mia may no longer exist? That she must now be a different Mia, whether she likes it or not. A Mia who relies on the help of others. One who can't brush her teeth or tie her long hair into a ponytail alone, because the strength of her hands and the lack of dexterity no longer allow it. One who spends most of the day lying down because independent sitting is no longer possible. Lying down, staring at the ceiling, dreaming of a life she could have had. This life was hers yesterday and today it belongs to others. She, on the other hand, was delivered a life that came by express mail and was never ordered. Can I return it, she must ask herself. How do I get out of this?

I won't ask her all these questions. Not now, while she's still in the hospital, and I leave her alone with her thoughts when visiting hours end. Sometime later, I'll ask her. When it's time. When she's with me, and I can be her anchor.

"Hey, anything happening?" Tony asks Mia as we arrive in her hospital room around four in the afternoon, giving her foot a playful pinch.

Meanwhile, I open the windows to let in some fresh air. It's stuffy in the room. After all, it's nearly ninety degrees today. A very warm start to September. The stench of urine in the neurology ward corridor was barely bearable when we arrived. As on every day, several carts stood outside the patient rooms.

Each with freshly changed full urine bags hanging from them. Yellow in all shades, I thought at the sight. Depending on how much each patient has had to drink, I concluded. Fortunately, here in Mia's hospital room, it's just hot, with a hint of disinfectant and oranges in the stale air.

"Nah, nothing's happening," Mia replies. "But Doctor Harper says it'll be fine. He must know," she adds with a smile.

"Mom brought you a smoothie," Tony responds, grinning at her and then at me.

"It's really tasty. No need to look so skeptical, Tony. With banana and all. Tastes really good," I explain to Mia, relieved that the coffee cup isn't transparent and her noticeable red smoothie isn't visible. "You can try it later. It'll definitely help."

"Yeah, okay, just put it somewhere on the nightstand so it doesn't spill," Mia asks me, "and then we need to quickly write an email. Guess what? I got the job. They want me," she tells me, her face beaming with excitement.

"Oh, really?" I respond hesitantly, not quite sure what to say. Of course, I understand her joy. I just wonder what sense it makes to take the job now when working obviously won't be possible for her in the near future. After all, she can't even move, let alone get up and do a student job. What's more, we don't know how long this condition will last.

On the other hand, I can't bring myself to dissuade her from taking the job right here and now. To talk her out of it so she changes her mind on her own.

"Let me see," I reply, taking her phone to read the email. "They even attached a contract. Have you seen the attachment? You're supposed to start in fourteen days," I add as I examine the contract. "Do you think... that's doable?" I look at her and feel embarrassed by my question, which isn't really a question. Rather, I want her to understand how unlikely it is for her to be back on her feet by then.

Her sight touches me. The hope in her eyes. And then the realization of her actual situation. Feeling tears welling up in my eyes, I turn away briefly to grab a chair. Meanwhile, Tony catches my gaze and says, "I'll go grab some coffee."

"Mia," I whisper as I sit beside her bed. "You can always take the job later. Rest first. That's more important now. Look, they must have been impressed by your interview if they're sending you a contract right away. That means even if you decline now, you can still contact them later."

"No, Mom, I can't. The company needs someone now, not later," she says, and I notice the first tear in her eyes.

I stroke her cheek.

"But what should I do," she adds softly. "Look at me. I'm here in diapers, can't even brush my teeth on my own. I understand that taking the job won't work. But… I was so happy."

"I know, sweetie. I'm sorry," I say.

"Mom, you have nothing to apologize for. You're right. Just send them an email saying I found something else, and that's it."

"Okay," I reply, unlocking her phone's screen when I notice three letters in the top left corner and gulp.

Ben. An unread message from Ben blinks almost imperceptibly on the phone screen. Not him again, I think, feeling anger rising within me. What does he want from her now? I thought that was over for good.

Maybe I should just delete the message. It must have arrived just now. I certainly didn't notice it earlier. I would have seen that, I ponder, with a thousand thoughts racing through my mind as I begin typing what I think would be the response to the employer.

"Can you read the email out loud when you're done? So we can see how it sounds and if we need to change anything," Mia asks me in the meantime.

"Sure, sure, just wait a moment. I'm just drafting it," I say.

So she's still in touch with him, I realize, and the mere thought makes it hard to swallow. I watch her from the corner of my eye. She's become thin. Her legs and arms are completely emaciated. Before this relapse, she was already very slim and hardly had any appetite because of the problems with this guy, Ben. Now there's nothing but skin and bones, no muscle mass left. She certainly doesn't need Ben's mind games during this time. His constant psychological manipulations have already taken their toll on her.

On one hand, I deeply despise Ben for that and don't want him to bother Mia here in the hospital. On the other hand, deleting a message from her phone would be a breach of trust. I can't do that.

So, what do I do with this message now? I have to make a decision in the next five seconds so she doesn't notice. Delete it or not? Open it and wait for her reaction?

Then my gut decides. No, I'll leave this message as it is. Mia is twenty-four. She makes her own decisions. And as her mother, I have to live with that. Whether I like it or not. Even if it means leaving the hospital today with a heavy heart and not sleeping for the next few nights. Once again, all because of that guy. Ben.

Thursday, 5th and last day of plasmapheresis

"It's already Thursday," Tony remarks as we reach the hospital grounds, like we do every afternoon. "And again, no parking spot available," he adds, annoyed.

"Well, you go park then. I'll stop by the bakery near the pharmacy. Mia wanted something sweet. Should I bring you something too?" I reply, stepping out of the car.

"Any pastry will do. Preferably sweet," he answers as I retrieve my handbag and the bag with Mia's dinner from the back seat.

"Okay. Then I'll see you at Mia's in twenty minutes. By the time I get back from the bakery, you can head up to the ward. And try not to take too long to park."

I grin at the thought of how long it might take him this time to find a parking spot, to snug his beloved car into the right spot. Not here, not there.

There's always some reason it won't work, I think, still smiling to myself as I walk across the gravel from the parking lot towards the bakery. About twenty minutes, I said. That should be about right for the distance across the sprawling hospital grounds. If I don't end up standing forever in line at the bakery, I ponder, simultaneously wondering why I didn't give Tony the bag with the food. Pretty stupid to lug it around now.

But then again, everyone here is carrying some bag or tote, I think, watching the people passing by. Adults, children, young, old, tall, short. And they all have a destination. I suddenly view all these people with different eyes. How small we all are and how dependent our bodies are on all the arts practiced in this great factory.

Essentially, we're like game pieces needing occasional refurbishment, repair, or overhaul. Then, we must come here. To the factory, called the hospital. In this moment, I ponder how rudimentary our bodies truly are. They're not perfect if they don't function flawlessly. At least imperfect enough that at some point in life, one must avail themselves of this factory's services. Some sooner, some later. We are vulnerable. Imperfect, and above all, not omniscient.

It's only for this reason that Mia, since that fateful Friday nearly two weeks ago when she was admitted here, has made no progress. Nothing has changed in her condition. What kind of factory is this, I still wonder, as the bakery clerk brings me back to reality.

"What can I get for you?"

In the evening, around midnight, I lie in bed unable to sleep. I can hear the television from the living room through the bedroom door. Tony must have dozed off on the couch, I think, or else the program wouldn't be so loud. Briefly, I consider waking him to join me in bed, but then I discard the thought. Somehow, I need these moments alone in bed at night. It allows me to replay the afternoon in my mind. So, I turn off the bedside lamp and stare at the ceiling in the dark.

Indeed, it took me a good thirty minutes this afternoon to finally reach the neurological ward after my bakery errand. Just as I was about to open the door to Mia's hospital room, a passing nurse called out, "She's been moved to another room last night."

Like an electric shock, fear surged through my arms in that moment. Moved, what does she mean? Why moved? But when I rushed to the next room and heard Mia and Tony laughing behind the closed door, I felt immensely relieved.

The night before, one of Mia's roommates had been transferred to another ward. And the seventy-three-year-old Maria had been discharged this morning, Mia later explained, just before a nurse served her dinner on the nightstand. But she wouldn't mind being alone in a room either. Doctor Harper had ordered it so she wouldn't have to stay with the really old and seriously ill patients in one room. I couldn't quite share her joy, I thought, watching her laboriously eat my homemade risotto with a spoon. She couldn't manage soup alone, I noticed immediately. Although she can use her hands somewhat, fine motor movements are impossible. What if she scalds herself, falls out of bed, or needs something that's not within immediate reach of her hospital bed? She can't walk, after all. So far, I've always relied on Maria to help her where possible. Even the emergency call button doesn't quite reassure me. Especially since Mia told us about today's lunch disaster. Her diaper was full, but the summoned nurse kept putting her off. There was just too much going on, she was told, and she needed to be patient. With a full diaper. She didn't touch her lunch, she continued. How could she, feeling so miserable in that state? No one could eat like that.

"Seems like they prefer me with constipation," she joked, and we laughed.

In the early afternoon, she exchanged text messages with Grandma. You know how Grandma texts, she explained with a smile.

Well, I think now as I lie in bed, it's a pity my mother doesn't have a smartphone. Then the two of them could see each other. But modern phones haven't reached her post-war generation yet, and I'm glad she can make and receive calls and read and write texts. That's enough. I smile at the thought, but suddenly the sound of an incoming text message startles me. Now, just after midnight? My heart races. A jumble of thoughts swirls through my mind. In seconds, I imagine the worst scenarios. Something has happened to her. The hospital is messaging me first to help me cope with the news. But who does such a thing? Who sends text messages to patients' families in the middle of the night? Meanwhile, I grab the phone from the nightstand and squint at the screen. I haven't put on my glasses. Without contacts or glasses, I feel almost blind. I still marvel at this after forty-four years, even though I should know better by now. However, the dread of what I might discover on my phone screen stops me from reaching for my glasses. Instead, I hold the phone two inches from my eyes and open a video attachment that Mia seems to have sent me.

Immediately, I recognize Mia's hospital bed. She must have recorded the video herself because the phone camera only shows her outstretched legs on the light blue hospital sheet, filmed from her perspective. How thin she has become crosses my mind immediately. Her legs are just skin and bones. And yet, her toenails are painted pink, I notice, and I smile. I know how much it means to her, even in this situation. But why is she sending me a video of her outstretched legs, I wonder the next moment. I squint to discern exactly what I apparently don't see in the semi-darkness of her bedside lamp. No one else seems to be in her room because it's quiet. Not even Mia says anything. Something that could explain to me what this recording is for.

And then the unbelievable happens. In slow motion, she pulls both legs toward her body until they are bent. What I see is so unbelievable that I watch the video over and over again. Tears stream down my face as I close my eyes in the dark and cry softly with relief. She actually moved her legs. My prayers have been answered.

Mia will walk again.

– Chapter 9 –

September 2018

A warm late summer day in Maplewood. Mia and I are sitting in a park that transitions into the nearby forest area. I'm on one of the wooden benches, Mia in her wheelchair. With our eyes closed, we let the afternoon sun warm our faces and listen to the cheerful chirping of birds. Nearby, a stream murmurs, and there's a scent of fresh forest soil. And sulfur.

"Well, you really have to get used to this stench," I explain, wrinkling my nose. "It smells disgusting."

"Thermal baths, you know," Mia replies, laughing. "It smells like this all day, everywhere. But you get used to it. After almost three weeks, I hardly notice it anymore."

Yes, in Maplewood, you inevitably get used to everything offered here. Even to the MS-Rehabilitation Center where Mia has been staying for seventeen days now to get back on her feet.

When we arrived at the Rehabilitation Center, I had to take a deep breath. A building that seemed to be from the nineteenth century awaited us with its seemingly endless corridors. Pale green walls and low-hanging ceilings made it feel like the place was crushing us from above. Countless white doors on either side seemed to lead to patient rooms. Every few meters, old white iron beds seemed to lean against the walls, as if waiting for new patients to arrive. Patients who couldn't possibly belong to modern times, as they didn't fit the overall picture. Even the cheerful hustle and bustle in the corridors didn't seem to fit into this image. Nurses and orderlies walking around. Smiling, joking with patients in the corridors. A shout here, a helping arm there. Patients in wheelchairs. Without legs, without arms, with crutches, limping, yet seemingly happy. Radiating a contentment that initially seemed out of place but then brought me a comforting sense of well-being.

If only the unbearable stench wasn't there, I thought. At first, Tony and I assumed it was the smell of urine wafting from the communal toilets into the hallway. But soon, we realized it was even worse. A combination of urine and sulfur. It felt like that foul odor was penetrating every fiber of my being through my nose. So, this is where my daughter would spend the next three weeks, I thought, looking around.

Because that's what Doctor Harper decided unexpectedly after nearly three weeks in neurology. I actually thought he would finally discharge Mia home. Two weeks of plasmapheresis, one week of observation. That should be enough. Until one afternoon during visiting hours, Mia broke the news to Tony and me.

"I'm supposed to go to MS-rehab. And it's happening the day after tomorrow."

"What do you mean, you're supposed to go to MS-rehab?" I asked, puzzled. "We didn't hear anything about this."

Everything was already arranged. Set in stone. Doctor Harper explained to her during rounds that it was important to advance Mia's recovery immediately with appropriate rehabilitation. Yes, she said, if he thought so, it was probably the best. So, the access tube in her throat was removed before the ambulance departure, which was meant for emergencies. They had left it in place for several days after the plasmapheresis in case another round of blood washing was necessary, the head nurse explained. And so, on the morning of September 13th, off we went to the Maplewood Rehabilitation Center. Single rooms, no stars, but full board. Mia sent me cheerful snapshots from the ambulance. However, the only thing I could make out was the interior ceiling of the ambulance. But clearly, the cellphone picture was meant to amuse me. Mia, the joker. Look, she seemed to be telling me, now it's off to the luxury vacation.

Unfortunately, I didn't have the opportunity to discuss the new therapy approach with Doctor Harper regarding these B-cells and that annoys me. Suddenly, everything had to happen so quickly. After all, getting a therapy spot in MS-rehab wasn't easy. Some patients wait for months for approval of their MS-rehab application. So, we should consider ourselves lucky.

Once the MS-rehab was decided, it had to start immediately. A day before the medical transport, Tony then told me his parents need help with the grape harvest. Well, I thought, like every year. But right now, it would have helped if he didn't go to the island during this time. Truth be told, I'm angry about it, but I keep my mouth shut. On top of that, Maplewood is ninety car minutes away from our place, and I don't have a driver's license. If I wanted to visit Mia in the next three weeks, I'd have to come by bus.

So, the evening before Mia's arrival at the MS-rehab, I sat down at the computer and searched for the best bus connection to Maplewood. Whatever 'the best' may mean, I thought, as I looked at the very limited transport options. Because there's no direct bus connection. Just getting here today took me over two and a half hours: first taking the subway from home to the main station, then catching the bus to the nearest city to Maplewood, which, by the way, only runs every two hours. Then, hopping on another bus through all the surrounding villages. However, all of this is worth it now that I see the sparkle in Mia's eyes as we sit here in the park.

It wasn't easy for me to push her out of her room through the corridors and onto the street and into the park. Not because I couldn't handle her lightweight, but because it's a wheelchair she's sitting in. Yet, I'm surprised by this familiar feeling as I push, something I wasn't expecting. Familiar because it's not the first time I've pushed my child in something. Only, it used to be a stroller. Her beloved stroller, which was our companion until she turned three during walks, shopping, outings in nature, visits to grandma and grandpa. This familiarity now consoles me over the fact that this isn't really what's supposed to be happening. She should be walking, not sitting in this wheelchair.

Fortunately, since her arrival at the MS-rehab clinic, she's been working hard to ensure that it doesn't stay that way. From the very first hour, she diligently practices in the physio room to become the person she once was. However, some exercises are only possible in a modified form, she tells me during my visits to the MS-rehab. For instance, riding the stationary bike can only be managed while sitting in the wheelchair and pedaling. For a start, that's already a significant progress, she thinks. Until recently, she couldn't even move her legs, let alone think about pedaling bicycle pedals. Now she fights her way back to life every day with small steps, through physiotherapy on the mat in the common room, cycling, and other exercises, all with the life she envisions firmly in sight. A life where she can do everything that will make her independent again. Her tireless optimism, which amazed me again a few days ago, plays a significant role in this. Suddenly, she had the idea to post a picture on social media.

"From the MS-rehab program?" I asked in disbelief.

"Sure, why not. Just do my makeup a bit, I'll sit on the bed so the wheelchair isn't visible, and take a selfie. No one will recognize the background. Hashtag rehab," she adds, and around her mouth, I see the mischievous smile that's so typical of her.

Yes, I thought, looking at her, she refuses to be beaten down. However, it's not always easy for me to stay positive constantly, even though I keep reminding myself to look forward.

Sometimes it's just difficult, and I find myself in situations that remind me of how she's really doing. Situations where I'm not immediately aware of how we must appear to others. I myself then think she's doing great, considering the condition she was in just a few weeks ago. But others only see Mia in the wheelchair. Just earlier, I found myself in one of these situations as we drove past the "Sunshine" café on our way from the MS-rehab clinic to this park, and suddenly I felt pitying glances behind me. The looks from passersby and café patrons made it clear to me that they felt sorry for a mother pushing her young daughter around the grounds. After all, everyone else here is much older, and at Mia's age, this fate is even harder to bear. "No one wishes for that," was written over their heads.

I wanted to shout at them, "Hey, don't look so pityingly. This is only temporary. She's already taking a step or two. It won't stay like this!" But I just looked away, pushing Mia along the gravel path into the park. I have my own prognosis and don't need this pity. Because I know better, I thought, feeling almost like a defiant child as I pushed her into the park.

Now, as we sit here in the sun, chatting away, that feeling has long faded. For the first time in weeks, I sense something akin to relaxation. Even though our conversations delve into topics we've been avoiding, like the new academic year starting in October. Hoping for a swift improvement in her health, Mia hadn't wanted to discuss returning to studies in recent weeks.

But now we know that a return to university this year isn't feasible. She can't walk more than two steps, is incontinent, and wouldn't even be able to take notes in lectures because her hand motor skills won't allow it. Even if she could hold a pen, the tremors in her hands would make writing impossible. These truths are unavoidable—and no longer deniable. So, I'll have to apply for a hiatus from the university on her behalf. Even though her disappointment is written all over her face, there's currently no other way out.

She can resume where she left off next late summer. But for now, it's about relearning the basics of daily life. Walking properly, eating alone, showering, and much more.

She took the first step in that direction on the second day of her arrival when she insisted on not wearing diapers anymore. A commode was needed instead.

"Now I have a nice little single room with a sink and a private toilet," she joked earlier.

Although 'nice' hardly does justice to the description I'd give this room. I'd call it more of a breeding ground for bacteria. After seeing the room, barely seven square meters on the first day, I returned half an hour later armed with cleaning supplies from the local convenience store. Spartan and tasteless, furnished with a cot, a small wardrobe, a table, a chair, and a sink. And to top it off, dirty. You can't recover from illness in a place like this, I thought while scrubbing away. Today, she has her own bedding from home, a warm blanket, and basic amenities like a soap dispenser in the room. At least that gives me hope she won't catch any more bacteria here.

What I can't scrub away with cleaning products, however, is what this illness must have done to her soul. Her friends only reach out sporadically now, she tells me. She doesn't like to talk about it, I can see that, but it needs to be said. I know what it must be like for her. Even I haven't felt understood by my friends in the past weeks and months. At the beginning of the diagnosis, during chats at the café or through text messages, there were inquiries about how Mia was doing. But the initial concern has evidently given way to restraint.

Often, I wonder about the reason. Is the fear that something as ominous as an illness could one day creep into their secure lives so great that they'd rather keep their distance? As if those of us whose lives have been touched by illness are contagious. As if merely talking about it could bring some of it into their lives. As if it could all rub off on them.

Grandma is the only one who writes to her regularly, she says. Of course, it's not the same as seeing each other, but for now, she'll settle for that. Since Mia's situation, my mother has been suffering from heart problems and needs to rest. A visit to Maplewood is out of the question. That's why Mia's current connection to the outside world is solely through her phone. To a world that, after three weeks in neurology, seems far too loud, too colorful, and too crowded, she tells me now in the park. You have to get used to all these impressions again. There wasn't much to see and hear in the hospital. Always the same doctors, nurses, caregivers. The same sounds and smells. And then there were the thoughts in her head. About the future. About what comes next. When she can expect this B-cell therapy and what it will actually do for her.

Yes, and then there are thoughts about the past. About a lost love. Josh. How much she had hoped there would be a future for both of them. But things turned out differently. It's been almost two years since their breakup, and she still bears the pain of it. He never reached out again after that day in December. Since she ended it all on her phone, what he could no longer give her. Comfort and understanding. Often, I wonder why she had to end up with Ben after that relationship. He was supposed to be a comfort, she tells me now, as the sun slowly disappears behind the trees in the Maplewood forest while we're still sitting in the park. He was supposed to console her through the time she still needs to lock away Josh somewhere in her heart. Invisible yet always present. Far from her feelings. That's why she endured Ben's mistreatment. Just to not be alone during this time.

I know all too well that she longed for something that no longer exists. She wanted everything to be like it used to be. A boyfriend who made her feel like a part of something every day. A sense of unity where there's only 'us'. Where you plan everything together. Especially the future. Dreams that you make come true together. Far from the expectations and wishes of others. In a life that seems so colorful and full of happiness, that only that one person takes center stage, because you can't live without him. Not for a single hour, not for a minute.

Of course, in hindsight, I feel validated in my gut feeling and my fears about Ben. But what good does it do me? I wish she hadn't had to go through all of this. Even though the day has finally come when she explains everything to me.

At this moment, I wonder why she's still texting this Ben, knowing he's not good for her. However, I don't inquire further. After all, it would imply that I must have seen the text message on her phone recently. That is why I stay silent, as I often do, and hope for a swift and definitive end to her relationship with Ben.

October 2018

I love October on the island, as our little village gradually winds down, preparing for the end of the tourist season. During this time, the scent of fermenting grapes drifts from the wine cellars in the narrow streets of the old town. Local vintners create full-bodied wines from their laborious grape harvest. Whether for personal use or to earn a bit of extra money. It doesn't matter as long as it's good, and old Joseph and Anthony, old school friends from days gone by, compete to see who can make the best wine. Hoping their wine will be declared the best in the village this year, and that the entire village takes note.

Here, at last, is a place of stillness, where the soul finds its center again. Among the pine forests, where their fragrance mingles with the ocean, filling the air with a fresh burst of life. Worries and fears are like locked-away relics in this place, resting somewhere to remain silent. Because there's no room here for sickness and everything that didn't let us breathe in the past months. Things that choked us, threatened to suffocate us.

Three days after Mia's discharge from Maplewood, we went to the island with Tony. Each to their own parents' house, as we always do and like during our stays here. This year, however, Mia and I are staying at our vacation home for the first time. As I swing open the garden gate on the day of our arrival, I ponder the passage of summer in our absence. The garden, once meticulously tended, now lies wild, with the summer's warmth giving way to the gentle touch of the autumn sun.

And I love it. The shorter days, the cooler nights, and the tranquil seclusion amidst nature. Most of all, I revel in the fact that Mia can now enjoy this place under her own power. Because despite arriving at Maplewood in a medical transport, she bid farewell to the nurses and caregivers with crutches after three weeks. "This is genuine happiness," I mused at that moment. This is what it feels like. Genuine bliss.

Today marks exactly sixteen days and nights since we arrived on the island, relishing every moment. Often, I catch glimpses of Mia and can scarcely believe that we're simply sitting here on the terrace, sipping our cappuccinos in the afternoon sun. How fortunate I am, I think to myself, and smile. She's even wandering through the house now, though leaning on the walls for support. But who cares when she moves so independently and freely. She's still thin, however. We're working on that, even though her appetite hasn't been the same since this setback. It's a struggle, but occasionally I manage to coax her into eating that extra morsel, hoping it will help her gain a little more weight.

Our days unfold in our own rhythm, which might seem monotonous to others. Yet, it's this very monotony that helps us ease back into an everyday life where Mia finds her place. An everyday life where she brushes her teeth sitting on the edge of the bathtub in the morning by herself. Where she makes it to the toilet on her own, despite the urgency and the need for speed. A routine where she dresses and undresses herself, manages her utensils, and doesn't spill soup or rice all over the place.

But regaining these abilities doesn't happen overnight. There is no snapping of fingers, no skipping, no writing, no running, no standing on one leg, no getting up without trembling limbs. And yet, she's doing well. She walks, she sings, she laughs, she jokes. It almost feels like it used to be. Like before this summer, when everything was still going as it should. Every small step forward fills her with indescribable joy.

"Look, I'm brushing my teeth while standing."

"Look, this time I didn't hold onto the walls the whole time."

"Look, I'm coming down the stairs arm in arm without stumbling."

Until that one day. It must have happened overnight, I think, as I watch her one morning on the way from the living room to the bathroom. Is she walking slightly bent forward or is it just my imagination, I wonder. Somehow, it looked different yesterday. Well, maybe she has back pain from all the walking around the house, I reassure myself. Yes, that must be it, I think, feeling somewhat relieved, as I prepare breakfast.

In the evening, I notice a scene that makes me pause again, but I don't bring it up with Mia. That duck-like walk. The butt sticking out, the arch of her back more pronounced than usual. And again, she walks slightly bent forward. What's going on? I want it to disappear immediately.

However, nothing disappears. In the days to come, I observe hourly how all the painstakingly learned habits seem to slowly fade away. Like rewinding a cassette tape. Small glimpses give me hope that it's just because of the weather. That she slept poorly. Missed her vitamins. Or simply had a bad day. We all have those sometimes. Does it mean having a bad day when suddenly one leg gives out, I wonder on the other hand. No. I know all too well what will come next. What we should brace ourselves for again. Because within very short time—it may be four, five, or six days—we can no longer make the journey from the couch in the living room to the bed in the room. So far, I could still help her walk.

In the evenings after watching TV, leaning against the walls on one side, arm in arm on the other, shuffling in tiny steps just in socks through the hallway. No slippers. After all, she could get snagged on something with her foot. Every little bump on the floor becomes an insurmountable obstacle. A carpet, a door threshold becomes a risk of falling.

"Come on, I'll call Tony. He'll be here in five minutes and carry you," I suggest, but she doesn't want to. We'll manage it, is her ever-constant reply. So, I stay silent. And the next day, I fetch a big blanket from the closet for her to lie on.

"It's the only way, Mia. You lie down. Here's a pillow. And I'll pull you from the living room over to the bedroom."

And … we laugh. A laughter so liberating that I have to stop halfway to wipe the tears from my eyes. She puts on her amused face and sings as if this were a boat ride across the sea.

"Stop messing around now," I half-heartedly scold her and continue pulling her through the hallway to her bed.

There, I sit down on the floor next to her, and we look at each other.

"Kilimanjaro," I say and we burst out laughing.

The bed is a mountain to conquer. So, I hoist her onto this mountain with all my strength.

November 2018

The return trip from the island to the city couldn't be more stressful. We have a few hours ahead of us in the car after finally leaving the ferry crossing behind us. Mia is lying on the back seat with a pillow and a warm blanket. There's no other way because she hasn't been able to sit since last week. Every attempt to sit her upright makes her collapse sideways. Her legs are completely paralyzed and also keep stiffening up, so even lying down in the back of the car is a challenge. Tony quickly got her a new pack of adult diapers from the pharmacy before today's departure. A walk to the bathroom hasn't been possible for many days now. Mia and I quickly realized this after her body suddenly stopped even the last remaining functions.

For days, Tony would carry her from bed to the living room couch in the morning and back again in the evening. I took care of everything else. Because I'm her mother. Although Mia kept apologizing for me having to do this. Especially the diaper part. Number 1 is manageable, but then there's number 2. Yes, number 2 is different. As recently as June, she was still able to do at least that part on the toilet. But now, even that's no longer possible.

"Mia, I'm your mother. I don't want you to apologize. I love you, and I would do anything for you."

How else can I explain to her that a mother just does everything. No matter what it is. Everything. The constant calls and emails to Doctor Harper are certainly among the smaller things that come with it. As Mia's health deteriorated again more and more rapidly, I became downright panicked.

"What are we supposed to do now?" I asked Doctor Harper on the phone. "And when is this B-cell therapy finally going to start?" I pressed, not realizing how much my voice was trembling. Out of anger at this whole mess with the hospital's medical board.

Because now they're the ones deciding, not the health insurance, Doctor Harper explained to me. This time, the medication has to be paid for out of the hospital's budget. That's all well and good, but someone needs to do something about it, I explained. Her arms and legs are paralyzed, she experiences double vision in her right eye, wears diapers, has muscle cramps at night, and lies there unable to move. Her whole body is numb, I explained. From the sole of her foot to her face. Even her tongue and gums. This can't go on like this, I said to him.

But Doctor Harper only replied that we should come to the hospital first. To the emergency room, as usual. "Yes, as usual," I thought bitterly.

The green complex of buildings now almost feels reconciling to me. Mia has spent so much time here in recent months. Involuntarily and without being asked. In a way, forced into it. Still, this familiarity helps me now, as our path leads us here again day after day. Through the main entrance into the hall-like foyer with the orange benches, quiet in the afternoons. No patients ask for directions at the reception, passing their referrals through the opening in the plexiglass. No one walks around, sits, or waits. It's quiet, like every afternoon. To the left of the reception, you turn to go through a long corridor with light blue flooring. At this time of year, the warm heating air overwhelms you. That's why there's always a window slightly open on the right. At the end of the corridor is the cardiology waiting area, where patients wait to be called behind a glass door. Some stand, impatiently pacing in front of the entrance. Or they sit on the few benches. Past the coffee machine and the trash can with the brown bag, a wide staircase from cardiology leads to the second floor. You could take the tiny elevator for a maximum of three people, which doesn't fit a wheelchair. Or you could take the freight elevator right across, mostly used by hospital staff to transport the large meal carts. As soon as the freight elevator door opens, the smell of warm food hits you.

But we take the stairs. As usual. Because movement keeps me from dwelling on my thoughts. On the stairs we encounter some familiar faces. A male or female nurse here and there. They greet us with a brief nod or smile. It's come to this, I think. They know us. Unfortunately.

Doctors are rarely seen here in the afternoon. The morning rounds on the ward have long been over. It's not until the next morning that busy white coats will be bustling around here again.

On the second floor, the large glass door to Neurology awaits us reliably. The same bell. The same nurses who see us from afar and open the door for us. The same smile.

"Hello, there you are. What lovely thing do you have with you this time? Mia is surely waiting."

As soon as we step into the neurology corridor, familiar smells and sounds surround us.

That's what this hospital feels like. Just last year, this place was a source of dread for me. Or rather, a place of constant apprehension, where you just want to flee. Just get out, close the door, and be gone. Today, I not only know whether Nurse Susan is on this shift or the afternoon shift, and when Nurse Tom will be back. But I'm familiar with all the routines, gestures, conversations that take place in Mia's hospital room. Every day, I observe the same routine.

And it gives me stability. It gives me the feeling that they know what needs to be done to make Mia better. And it also includes corticosteroids. Too many, I keep thinking. Especially in such a short time. This must be the third or fourth time this year. But what choice do we have? In my desperation, I still hope for the miraculous effects of this treatment. Even though I know they no longer work for Mia. They want to try it anyway, they say.

But why do the doctors seem so puzzled during the morning rounds, as Mia often describes? She asks about the treatment plan. But she never gets a clear answer. Instead, she feels like the doctors are at a loss themselves. Only the B-cell therapy is an option. However, this topic is carefully avoided during the morning rounds, Mia says.

We need certainty, I keep thinking. We need to rely on her getting this therapy. And above all, I want to know when we can expect the therapy.

That's why two days after Mia's readmission to the Neurology ward, I request a meeting with Doctor Harper. I briskly make my way to his office on the ward, feeling almost anxious. To the outside world, I surely appear assertive. The doctors, nurses, and orderlies must think, "Here comes that mother again," whenever they see me. Why doesn't the daughter ask herself? A twenty-four-year-old should be able to find out information for herself. Without her mother constantly interfering and bombarding them with questions. These thoughts are clearly written in the head nurse's expression whenever I approach her.

No one seems to understand the emotional state Mia is in. So it's not surprising that as her mother, I sometimes have to take the lead. Otherwise, we'd be completely in the dark about the progress of her therapy and everything that comes with it. Even the side effects of all these corticosteroids go unmentioned. I almost get the impression they're instructed to reveal as little information as possible about them. "Just if asked, Nurse Susan. Otherwise, please don't tell the patients anything." And upon asking, the odd snippet of information is reluctantly shared. Perhaps just to placate me for a while. At least for a little while. Or is it easier to leave this part to the doctors? "Please ask the doctor. I'm afraid I can't provide you with that information."

So, that's how I come across. Assertive, and above all, annoying. Internally, though, I'm torn apart by fear of what Doctor Harper might say to me in his office.

He's already waiting for me outside his office, which is one floor below the Neurology ward.

"Go ahead and take a seat, I'll be right back," he says, pointing to a chair in the tiny room before stepping out into the corridor.

I settle into an office chair positioned in the middle of the room, realizing that I've never spent more than a minute here before. Usually, I just stood briefly in the doorway to ask him something. For the first time, I truly take in his office, feeling as though the room is speaking to me: "Look, this is Doctor Harper for real!"

I glance around. A room no larger than seventy-five square feet. Two desks sit side by side against the right wall. Two computers, two black office chairs. The left one is his workplace, I remember. The spot by the window with the stacks of files. A report seems to be open on his computer screen. I can't make out what's written there. Maybe it's Mia's report, I think, but I remain seated. After all, it could be another patient's report. I imagine how it would look if Doctor Harper suddenly walked in and found me staring at the screen. That would be embarrassing.

So, I sit here and let my gaze wander across his desk. Stacks of papers, pens, the usual. And then I spot a cup with a heart on it next to his keyboard. I wonder who it's from. From a woman, I think the next moment. The young, hip Doctor Harper, who always seems so cool. How did he win her over? Open, funny, maybe even playful? Quite different from here in the hospital, where he exudes competence and aloofness.

I glance out the window. It started raining earlier, and now the rain is coming down harder. Mia particularly loves autumn, it occurs to me. When she leaves the house in the morning in her autumn coat, running through the leaves to catch the bus. Always carrying her umbrella. A small one that fits in her bag. The one with the leopard print. She loves this rainy weather, the scent of winter approaching. When you never know what to wear in the morning because the sun might come out in the afternoon and you'll end up sweating. Layering. That's her thing.

I imagine her coming home in the afternoon. Her hair damp from the drizzle, smelling of her favorite shampoo. She takes off her brown ankle boots in the hallway, hangs up her coat on the coat rack, and sits down on the small bench in our foyer. To quickly eat something before leaving the house again because the day is far from over. Because there's still so much she wants to do today. What she's looking forward to. And now... now she's lying there, I think to myself, and my stomach tightens. After everything that happened to her in the months before this relapse, I shouldn't be surprised by this new setback. All the stress at work, then her studies. And Ben. At the thought that this condition could now be permanent...

"So, here I am," Doctor Harper interrupts my thoughts as he enters the office. Then he sits down at his desk and turns to me. "You wanted to talk to me."

"What happens now, Doctor Harper?" I ask him, and he must see the pain in those few words. Because I see him playing with a pen in his hand, apparently unsure how to phrase the next words for me.

"The medical board meets every Thursday. I've already been there three or four times. They're still deliberating," he answers, sounding hesitant to me.

"But will she even get this therapy?"

"She needs to get this therapy." He emphasizes the "needs" and looks me in the eye.

I fall silent, realizing in that moment how dire Mia's situation must be. Ever since her last stay before Maplewood, I've known about this B-cell therapy and had hoped it wouldn't be long after MS-rehab. But now, the prospect doesn't seem so certain anymore. I recall that "probably" he mentioned back in the summer. "Probably B-cell therapy." I was probably right. About the uncertainty in his words that I apparently interpreted correctly. Now, two months later, the therapy still hasn't been approved, and I wonder why. The same sentence circles in my head again and again. She can't stay like this. Although some doctors here seem to have a different opinion.

"Do you know what Doctor Winters said during the first visit two days ago when she saw Mia again? 'Why are you back again? Nothing's changed. You left us in this state,'" I complain to Doctor Harper now. "I don't know what she's thinking. In the meantime, Mia was even able to walk again after MS-rehab. She was doing well. You'd think Doctor Winters thinks there's nothing more to be done. But that's not true. There was improvement. And there will be again. She needs this B-cell therapy."

He looks at me and falls silent. Of course, he'll remain loyal to his colleague and won't comment on this incident. And yet

I want him and everyone else here to know that my daughter doesn't have to stay in this state just because they don't give her a chance.

"Doctor Harper, the patient up there in Neurology isn't just anyone, some patient XYZ. That's my child," I explain, my voice trembling, pointing my finger upward. "Some people may not care what happens to her. But I care! I care how she spends the next sixty years of her life."

"I know," he replies, "I'll speak with all the neurology colleagues again before the medical board on Thursday. We're doing our best."

As I leave Doctor Harper's office a few minutes later, I wonder whether his last sentence was meant to reassure me or just placate me for the moment. Because after two years, we're back to square one. Starting over. We need a therapy.

December 2018

Ten days after my last conversation with Doctor Harper, Mia is discharged from the hospital. It feels like they're sending me home with a newborn. Strangely, on the day of her release, I'm struck by the same thoughts I had twenty-four years ago. Back then, as a twenty-year-old mother, I left St. Joseph's Hospital with my baby in a carrier, thinking, "Now I have to do this on my own. I hope I can manage it." Almost nostalgically, I reminisce twenty-four years later about how proud I was to embark on the journey of caring for my baby myself. Nursing, changing diapers, bathing, cuddling. And marveling. Spending the whole day marveling at this little wonder in her crib.

Today, Mia is an adult. Nothing and no one prepared me for this moment. Quickly, Mia, Tony, and I arrive home on the day of her discharge, needing to navigate the new situation within our own four walls. There were no instructions, guidance, or even advice on how to care for Mia in the hospital. After Tony carried her from the car to the apartment on the first floor, I hastily clear the way so he can lay her down on the couch. Fully bundled up for winter. I quickly take off her boots while Tony still holds her. Tony and she joke about how well he can carry her because she's so thin and how she must not gain weight. From now on, she declares with a laugh that she'll only eat burgers.

And in the next moment, she's lying there. Stretched out on the couch. Her arms and legs paralyzed, partially stiff. Now what? is my first thought. What do we do now, and, most importantly, how?

First, we decide that Mia will temporarily move out of her room and sleep with me in the parents' bedroom. Meanwhile, Tony will be accommodated in a dream of girly colors in her room. Among makeup utensils and university books. It may not be typical, but for us as a family, there's no long debate about it. We have to find solutions. After all the hospital stays and MS-rehab, Mia yearns for security and comfort. Especially since she can no longer manage simple things like turning over in bed at night. And from constantly lying on her back, she gets backaches. Not to mention my fear that she might develop bedsores, like many older patients in the hospital. So from now on, I have to be near her all the time. Whether it's day or night. Always there to help when she needs me.

Within a few days, the room change proves to be the right decision. Unexpectedly, the nightmares begin.

One night, she suddenly calls out, "Mom?" into the darkness of our bedroom.

"Yes, sweetie. I'm here. What happened?" I immediately snap on the bedside lamp, noticing her sweaty hair. "What's wrong, sweetie?" I ask, stroking her face.

"I thought the nurses were coming. There were loud voices. It felt like they were coming into the room in the morning to draw my blood." The terror on her face makes me realize the marks the long stays in the clinic must have left on her soul.

These marks cause a new distress during the nights. Spasms in her otherwise immobile legs. Suddenly, her legs bend with unexpected force, locking in a cramp, causing her to cry out in pain. As if enduring the nightmares wasn't enough. In nights that should have transported her into the world of dreams. Into a world free from suffering and pain. No longer trapped in her own body.

Feeling helpless about this additional symptom of the illness makes me do what's possible in the perplexing darkness of the night. I comfort her. I gently stretch her leg into the right position and massage it until she falls asleep again. What else can I do, I wonder. And why didn't the doctors tell me about it? They left me alone to discover what else might happen. Why on earth didn't anyone inform me that such spasms could occur?

And why wasn't something prescribed preventively. For every symptom, there's a remedy. Muscle relaxants that could spare her additional pain. Why didn't anyone tell me anything, I wonder, feeling a kind of anger. An anger that quickly dissipates, as another thought creeps into the darkness of the bedroom.

The question of what might be the true origin of these nightly cramps. Perhaps Mia's inner battle, I reflect in the next moment, as I listen to her breathing. A battle that only she knows and must fight alone. Like all of us. Because no one peers inside us. No one comprehends all the dormant fears and worries of our soul, hidden deep within us, each leading its own existence. And then the subconscious comes and exposes us in the night. Turns our innermost outward for a moment and lets us feel what we dare not feel. In a nightmare that must be unmasked to free ourselves from it.

Within a few days, we follow a certain routine, beginning with the morning diaper change in bed. Often, I wonder why no one gave me a tip before leaving the neurology department on how to best turn Mia onto her side. In the hospital bed with fold-down rails on both sides, it was apparently very easy.

But how do I manage that in our double bed at home? Every time I've grabbed Mia by the shoulder and hip to turn her onto her side, her paralyzed and stiff body rolls back onto her back like a sack of potatoes. So even changing the diaper becomes a challenge. Turning, lifting, and shifting. And Tony can't assist me with these tasks; after all, it's about the personal hygiene of an adult young woman. That doesn't make things any easier.

Suddenly, I recall the old trick of placing a rolled-up towel behind my baby Mia's back while she slept, to prevent her from rolling onto her back. Back then, there was a belief that sudden infant death syndrome was linked to sleeping on the back, and it was to be avoided at all costs. Now, more than twenty years later, that memory proves useful, although I would have preferred not to revisit it.

Like so many other things.

Dressing my adult daughter. Feeding her.

Her sight, which reminds me every day how her life has changed from that of a vibrant student to that of a dependent patient in just a few months. Each task serves as a daily reminder of that to me.

Particularly saddening, however, is the act of bathing. A soak in our corner bathtub is out of the question, as nothing in our apartment is wheelchair accessible. Even if Tony were to carry her to the tub, she wouldn't be able to sit in it. Because she cannot sit anymore.

I recall a nurse mentioning something about a wheelchair and an accessible shower. But such changes don't happen overnight. In an instant, the bathtub is gone, and an accessible shower appears. Not to mention, Mia doesn't want to hear anything about such renovations. Disabled. That's not her, and she doesn't want to be treated as such.

So, bathing must take place on the couch. A large turquoise plastic tub, steam rising from warm water, now sits beside me on the floor. On the coffee table, I lay out several washcloths to cleanse Mia. And once again, I find myself transported back to the time when she was still a baby. In the first days at home, I washed her like this. In a baby tub with plain water and a washcloth. Only my thoughts were different back then. And the emotions that this washing evokes in me today. Melancholy. Yes, melancholy settles on my chest as I wash Mia's body on the couch. Even though we laugh together during these moments, her helplessness is almost unbearable for me. The mere fact that she lies here on the couch, unable to care for herself, unable to move, tightens my throat.

"Are you cold? Should I turn up the heat a bit?"

"No, you don't need to. The water is warm. And if we do everything in order, it won't get cold."

I wash her in sequence so that her frail body doesn't get cold. First the upper body, then dress, and only then the lower body. That way, a part of her body is always clothed and warm.

"Tonight, 'The Voice' is on again. It's the battle rounds," I mention to Mia, hoping to steer our conversation to a lighter topic. "Who are you rooting for in the battle?" I ask as I continue to bathe her, attempting to maintain a sense of normalcy amidst the challenging circumstances.

"For the female voice," Mia replies, her voice carrying a hint of excitement despite the situation. Of course, she knows that this is just a distraction tactic. Not so much for her. But rather for me. After all, I'm the one who keeps getting caught drifting into thoughts that I evidently can't hide.

Sometimes, I fear Mia might hear my thoughts. As if I have to clamp my mouth shut to ensure I don't inadvertently voice them aloud. What if she doesn't recover? Or if the new therapy doesn't work either? How will she go on like this? It seems all of this is plainly written on my face. So, to escape from it, I steer our conversations toward other things.

Yet, I can't evade this here. Her frail arms beneath my hands as I bathe her. The bones protruding everywhere. The fact that there are no muscles left visible. Over the long months, it's evident that all the muscles in her arms and legs have vanished, and the extent of the illness is clearly visible on her body. How can I put on the facade of a cheerful mother when inside me, it's entirely different? Still, it seems cowardly to just accept things as they are.

Ultimately, it's Mia's life and her future at stake here. Not mine. That's why I have to remind myself time and time again that this will only be temporary. It won't be long until it gets better. Just one phone call away, where Doctor Harper informs me that the application for the B-cell therapy has been approved. And that's what we're waiting for, as one day after another slowly passes.

December days grow colder and shorter. When I open the windows during the day to air out the apartment, the scent of snow already wafts in, and for a fleeting moment, I feel a tiny bit of anticipation. A familiar feeling that reminds me of the upcoming Christmas season. All the wonderful preparations for the annual Christmas celebration. Beloved people, strolling through the Christmas market, fairy lights, candied apples.

But as suddenly as this wonderful feeling came, it vanishes again. Because this year, everything is different, I recall, as if I've woken up from a dream. There's no anticipation at all. No life as it once was. And then there's that dull sorrow again, leaving behind a feeling of unbearable powerlessness deep in my gut.

I close the window and leave that old world out there. Because my new world here in this apartment is a completely different one. Here, I wait day after day for that one phone call. Nothing else matters. Just that one call.

And in mid-December, it finally arrives. Doctor Harper calls me one morning just before eleven, as I'm filling the washing machine with dirty laundry in the bathroom.

"Is Mia nearby?"

"No, why?" I reply, checking if the bathroom door is locked.

"Listen, it seems like the medical board is going to reject the application. They'll be meeting again tomorrow, but…" He pauses.

"Yes?" I ask, my heart already racing wildly after those few words.

"I've spoken with Chairwoman Doctor Wright several times already. Just yesterday, in fact. Well, how should I put it, the approval doesn't look favorable," he continues, and I hear in his voice that he's searching for a way out.

"We should play another card," he adds. "Write a letter."

"A letter?" I ask, trying to quickly make sense of this statement in my head.

"Yes, a letter to the board. Request approval from a mother's perspective, so to speak. Tomorrow is Tuesday, the committee meets again. Like every week. Send the letter to my email by tomorrow morning at the latest. I'll be with my colleagues at the board by ten. Maybe they can be persuaded. If not tomorrow, then perhaps on one of the upcoming Tuesdays."

"But this feels so sudden." I pace back and forth in our tiny bathroom, look into the mirror, sit on the edge of the bathtub, then stand up again. "What exactly should I write?" I ask, although I'm already formulating sentences in my mind.

"Come up with something. One page is enough. Request without sounding accusatory. That could help us," he adds, and after a brief farewell, our conversation is already over.

Stunned by the reason for his call—a looming rejection—I sit back on the edge of the bathtub and stare at the phone screen for minutes on end. So I'm supposed to write a letter. One that apparently determines the future of my only child.

How does he expect me to do that, I wonder the same evening, as I sit in the dim light of my bedroom desk lamp with my laptop. Mia and Tony are watching our TV show in the living room. Under the pretext of an urgent translation that came in and needs to be done tonight, I now stare at an empty computer page. I'm exhausted. Yet, my nerves are on edge and won't let me rest. Still, I have to get this letter done now, I think, massaging my temples. With each passing minute, my headache worsens, as the nagging questions of how and what drive me crazy.

First, you need to organize your thoughts, I admonish myself then. Everything could depend on this. They've placed the fate of it all in my hands, without knowing how heavy this responsibility weighs. I am her mother. No one could care more about her recovery than me. How can Doctor Harper expect me to put that into words?

On the other hand, this letter gives me the opportunity to participate in the board's decision-making process. With my words, I could set something in motion in the minds of the members and achieve what I desperately want. Specifically, I want this B-cell therapy to no longer be a distant goal but to positively change Mia's life in the near future.

So how do I reach the board members, I wonder. Doctor Harper had cautioned me not to accuse the chairwoman in my letter. To choose my words carefully, avoiding any accusation, a prudent inner voice warns as I gaze out the bedroom window.

It's dark, and the street in front of our building is illuminated only by a streetlight. Snowflakes dance in the glow of the lamplight. I imagine one of the members, a fifty-something, wrapped in his warm winter coat, strolling along a shopping street, admiring the Christmas displays in the windows. After a long day at work, he's left the clinic and is now searching for Christmas gifts for his loved ones. He must already have a wife and two children at this stage of life. He cherishes the time with his small family, especially during the Advent season, looking forward to the upcoming holidays. So, he's a loving father who takes his role as a doctor in the medical board seriously and doesn't make hasty decisions. What words must I address to this father, I wonder.

But what if there's not a father sitting on the board? What if it's a doctor nearing retirement, who's spent his whole life living with his mother? An old bachelor, grimacing at the twilight of his days spent alongside a nearly ninety-year-old mother—certainly not the life he envisioned. She still makes his sandwiches daily for work at the clinic and eagerly awaits him in the evenings with warm pea soup and slippers by the window, ready to spend the night watching game shows on TV together. At what point must I confront this embittered man who's long since resigned himself to his own well-being and likely has little sympathy for the heartaches of others?

The chairwoman, I think in the next moment. That's who I need to address. She's a woman. Subconsciously if not consciously guided by emotions that should prevail in such matters of conscience. Because... well, because she's a woman. Isn't it scientifically proven that the female brain is an expert in emotions, I muse, spotting a young woman on the street outside our house. She's holding a little boy's hand, and I imagine they're on their way home from kindergarten. She's carrying his small backpack with some comic book hero emblazoned on it over one shoulder and seems impatient to me. The boy seems eager to revel in the snowfall, repeatedly letting go of her hand. But she wants to keep moving forward. "Come on, let's go home," she seems to be coaxing him.

In that moment, I wonder if the chairwoman might be a single mother. A woman who juggles work and motherhood every day. Plagued by the familiar guilt of every working mother, she likely wonders throughout the day what her child is doing. How his day at kindergarten is going, whether he's playing with other children or sitting alone in a corner. She contemplates all they'll do together once they're home in the late afternoon. After tending to the household chores.

And what they'll do over the weekend. Maybe they could go on a trip to the zoo or indulging in cotton candy at the Christmas market. Yet, even the most colorful plans and outings fail to suppress this guilt within her. It constantly gnaws at her, making her question whether she's living up to it all. The demands of her job as a doctor and chairwoman of the medical board weigh heavily, especially in a male-dominated world where no one cares if the child falls ill. It's a continuous struggle to prove herself. Because, after all, only performance matters. On the other hand, there's her own child, who should want for nothing. Especially not love and attention.

How should I address my plea to such a woman, or one similar to her? I must reach the right corner of her heart, one that momentarily sets aside the strict regulations of her position. Mia's future now hangs by a thread of my words, I realize in the next moment. If I choose the wrong ones… the thread could break. In the end, it might be a single word that tips the scale. A word I don't yet know, I think, and this thought fills me with renewed fear. One I must find in the sea of words, as everything now depends on this letter.

"Just start," I say aloud, though no one can hear me in the bedroom. "Just write, whatever comes. Anything is better than doing nothing."

So I write.

Esteemed Chairwoman,
esteemed members of the Medical Board,

I hereby request from you, as the mother of your patient Mia Madalena V., the approval for the B-cell therapy with the medication OC.

My only daughter, Mia, is twenty-four years old, and her young life has only just begun. Like any young person, Mia has dreams and aspirations in life. She studies, loves poetry, and is a very lively young woman.

However, Mia has now become a case requiring constant care due to the severe and prolonged deterioration of her health. She spends her days bedridden, paralyzed in her arms and legs, in diapers, and in pain, isolated from the outside world. Since her last hospitalization, her condition has been deteriorating noticeably.

With the approval of the B-cell therapy, you would be granting Mia the opportunity to continue her young life with dignity. This medication, available in your clinic, could offer her a life that every one of us wishes for our child.

I implore you not to deny Mia this opportunity.

With sincere gratitude,

Mother of the patient Mia Madalena V.

It's been over a week now since Doctor Harper presented my letter to the medical board, but there's been no response.

The more I've revisited my own words in these past days, the more awkward and clumsy they seem in hindsight. Could I have done better, I wonder at one moment. And at another, I imagine the chairwoman reading my letter. Which sentence, which word, might evoke in her what I hoped to achieve.

In my mind's eye, she sits at her desk in the clinic office shortly after receiving my letter, her gaze scanning over my lines. Initially, she merely skims through the few sentences, but then the final paragraph gives her pause. "A life that every one of us wishes for our child."

Just moments ago, what she read was just another desperate mother's letter. Suddenly, however, there's this word. Child. She understands that for the writing mother, it's not just about any patient whose well-being she's concerned about. It's about her child. The dearest person she has.

I imagine the chairwoman pausing briefly. She leans back in her office chair and removes her reading glasses. She still holds my letter in her hand, staring blankly into space for minutes. How can she reject such a request, she wonders, without compromising her own sense of morality? Without later having to wonder what would have become of this young patient if she had just approved the request. She knows all too well that this B-cell therapy offers such patients a possibly final chance to emerge from unexpected misery and still experience some of the happiness in life that undoubtedly belongs to them.

Now it's up to her alone. Though there are other board members, she knows her word is final and decisive. She doesn't sit in this chair for nothing. The chair of the chairwoman. A chair that grants her an often unwanted power that she sometimes wishes she could deflect onto someone else. Because some decisions weigh heavily. Decisions like these, she now thinks, looking again at my letter and sighing. What should she do? It's a week before Christmas.

These days, Mia sleeps a lot. Whether it's due to the infamous fatigue syndrome or her escape from the here and now, I can't say. I stay silent about it and let her sleep. Somehow, this time of sleeping gives me the chance to temporarily shed the constantly cheerful facade I put on for Mia. But as soon as she wakes up, I put it back on and wait for the same old question.

"Mom, what was the plan for today again?"

Yes, Mia has always liked plans. Now, however, her familiar and beloved routine is simply gone. University, work, boyfriend, friends. A daily rhythm that offered her security. Suddenly, it's all wiped out. A new routine is needed. One that I design for her to hold onto. Ultimately, we must not let the senselessness of our lives overshadow us. Excluded from the rest of the world, we live our own lives in six hundred ninety square feet. Even such a life must have shape. And Tony and I make sure of that every day. What's for lunch, which of our favorite shows is on TV today.

Independent physiotherapy exercises and the like are not yet feasible at the moment. But there's still passive activity. So that's also incorporated into our ongoing routine. Every day, Mia and I spend an hour massaging her arms and legs, moving them, propping them up, and stretching them out again.

"So your brain starts to remember the movement patterns again. We have to keep your body in good spirits so it doesn't forget all of this. Until the nerve pathways start functioning again," I explain to her with a smile.

Meanwhile, we mainly navigate from one TV show to another. The only bright spot is our favorite shows in the evening, which the three of us watch, comment on, and warm our hearts in the cozy atmosphere of a routine that gives us a bit of familiar comfort.

Of course, Mia knows about the letter by now. How could I hide something like that from her? She's an adult. I haven't read it to her, though. I explained it was a simple request for approval. But Mia probably senses my growing unease. Even my forced cheerfulness can't mask it. She knows me, and her finely tuned antennae pick up on when something's amiss with me.

And then there's the upcoming Christmas celebration. A mountain of tasks that seem insurmountable to me.

So, my Christmas preparations now feel like a dull execution of practiced routines in my mind. Tony is getting the tree. Normally, I'm the one who carefully selects the size and fullness of the tree. This year, I don't care. It can even be plastic, although I've always been strictly against putting such an artificial thing in our living room. I even consider leaving the decorating to him, but then I change my mind. I don't want Mia to see how I'm feeling.

Three days before Christmas Eve, I start decorating the Christmas tree with our ornaments. Just like every year. For almost twenty years now. And always with the same Christmas ornaments. Decorations I bought in New York in 1999. They've been bringing us a touch of Rockefeller Center and honking yellow taxis in the city's snowstorm ever since.

Mia is lying on the couch, watching me decorate. To drown out the chaotic thoughts in my head, I keep asking Mia where I should hang each ornament so that the colors are evenly distributed. But I can't escape these fragments of thought. They're gnawing at my nerves.

At one moment, I think the board can't possibly say no. Almost a surge of euphoria envelops me. I sense a wave of anticipation for the forthcoming confirmation from the clinic. In my mind, I'm already planning the next steps after starting the therapy. Ethan, our physiotherapist, will need to come back. Because as soon as Mia receives the medication, we'll need to start the initial exercises to remind her body of what it can do and where we want to go. Everything will be okay again. She'll walk again and participate fully in life as usual. At least, that's how I envision the next few months in this scenario.

But then there's this other voice. And this voice feels louder, more urgent, and echoes more in my mind. What if the application is rejected after all? What will I do then?

At night, I lay in bed, contemplating all the options I have left to obtain the medication. While Mia sleeps beside me in the darkness of the bedroom, a whirlwind of thoughts storms through my mind, keeping me from finding peace. My initial thought goes to my childhood home on the island. My parents worked their whole lives for it. In their early twenties, they began earning their money in a factory. This house is the symbol of their tireless diligence. But not only that. It's our home.

All the memories of my late father are embedded in it. In my mind's eye, I look back on the summers of my childhood in the seventies in this house. How much happiness we experienced here.

A happiness that became even more complete with Mia's birth. She loves the house. Grandpa's garden, where he always planted his tomatoes. Little Mia was allowed to help with the harvest.

"Look, this is how you easily pick the tomato. Just twist it a bit," Grandpa always explained to her.

Yet, in the next moment, I realize it's just a house. We'll all cope if it's gone. If other people find happiness in it. Because what good is the house to us now that Mia is ill? Nothing. Absolutely nothing. I stare into the darkness, wondering how many doses of the medication the money would cover if we decide to sell.

Not enough. Maybe three, four doses, the answer echoes in my mind. That's nowhere near sufficient. This treatment is just too expensive. I'd have to find another way to get money. But how?

A list of quick money-making opportunities runs through my mind. Becoming an influencer—that's what I should do, I realize then. Every post brings in money. If. Yes, if you have enough followers, I remind myself. Where will you get them from? Especially at the age of forty-something. Completely without "influence". What do you have to excel at? In the shortest time. I would have to become famous in the blink of an eye.

In my desperation, I briefly consider how I would need to change my appearance. Thousands of wild thoughts race through my mind. Even at my age, they all look so surgically altered and perfect. I can make myself look pretty too, but like that? So flawless from head to toe. Face, skin, hair, body. Always the perfect photo, from breakfast to dinner. I don't even have that much clothing, I think to myself and have to chuckle. All this perfection costs a ton of money, money that I could currently use much better. No, that won't work out quickly. I dismiss this flash of an idea.

Maybe I could bake or cook something. Sort of like a food influencer. That sounds more acceptable. I'd need good recipes. Something unusual. And I'd have to get a good camera. Then I'd have to set everything up and photograph it, edit the photos. In the end, I might even enjoy it, I start to imagine. But then a warning voice insists it's all nonsense. Mia needs the medication now. Immediately. Who becomes an influencer overnight, I remind myself. We need a tangible solution. Goodbye, influencer life.

Outside, a passing car briefly illuminates the ceiling, and I have a new idea. Crowdfunding. That's something I could try. Best on an international internet platform, where my plea will be seen. I've seen on TV how donations come together for people who really need it. It's worth a try. I could start researching the best website for it first thing tomorrow morning.

But then I'd have to upload photos of Mia, I think, and suddenly, unease washes over me. As far as I remember, such fundraising campaigns always use before and after photos. To make it clear to potential donors how dire the person's situation is. How wonderful their life once was and how utterly terrible it is now. So terrible that donations need to be collected. Usually, the person has no hair or is lying in a hospital bed, marked by an accident or a serious illness.

Does that mean I have to find one particularly beautiful and one particularly pitiful photo of Mia to present there? One showing her in the prime of her life as a carefree student. And the other from the hospital, hooked up to plasmapheresis, in diapers.

I don't want that. I don't want to put her on display like that. It just feels wrong, I think, and something rebels within me. How could I do something like that? Replace her former joy of life with an image of despair. That would be betrayal. Betrayal of her optimism and her daily courage to wake up in the morning, even though the world probably has nothing pleasant to offer her that day. No, you won't do that, I remind myself, dismissing this thought once again. There must be another way.

A cold wind greets me as I leave the house late in the afternoon, three days before Christmas. Just moments ago, I decided to pull myself together despite my melancholic state and finally get some Christmas shopping done. Tony stayed with Mia to take care of her. Outside, it's already getting dark, and a light blanket of snow has formed on the asphalt. I have to be careful not to slip on it with my non-winter-proof ankle boots. Our neighbor across the street seems to be baking cookies because there's a scent of cinnamon as I walk along the street. Well, the neighborhood is already getting ready for the Christmas celebration, I think, glancing at the windows lit up with fairy lights. It looks beautiful. Like every year.

After about five minutes of walking, I can already see the large fir tree at the bus stop in the distance. It's illuminated in gold. Not bad, I think. It gets louder here on the main street. You can hear the cars honking. Rush hour. People want to get home.

It reminds me of the time when I used to work in an office for one of the world's largest American corporations. When on such a pre-Christmas afternoon, after work, I would leave the large glass doors of the headquarters in the city center behind me and stroll through the main street to the subway. It felt similar. For a brief moment, I'm transported back to that carefree time thirteen years ago. Back then, I was so young and full of enthusiasm. I loved this Christmas atmosphere.

But now it makes me sad. This atmosphere. And Christmas in general. That's why we'll spend Christmas Eve and the Christmas holidays alone. We don't need a holiday that isn't one. Besides, Mia doesn't want to be seen like this, she told us on the first Sunday of Advent. Lying on the couch. In diapers. Immobile. Unable to sit at the festively set table and enjoy the feast with the family. She doesn't want that.

Nevertheless, I'll decorate our apartment somewhat festively and cook something for us. No cheerful acting in front of the family. No suppressed tears at the sight of others' normal lives. Scenes where I have to choose between the table and the couch. Between pretending to have a completely normal Christmas dinner and feeding my daughter on the couch. No, I don't want that either.

So our Christmas will be one where we're allowed to be introspective, without feeling compelled to conceal it. Of course, there will be laughter, jokes, and life lived in the moment on that day. But just different. In our own way, completely unromantic, I think now as I stand at the street corner waiting for the green light.

I observe the people passing by. Passing by, I think. They walk. Just like that. One foot in front of the other. Young, old, short, tall, fat, thin. Nothing can stop them. They don't even think about how walking works. And what it would be like if they couldn't do it anymore. If one foot suddenly refused to move in front of the other. What it would be like if this seemingly simple activity wasn't so simple anymore. Or even impossible. Game over.

But they just walk. And in that moment, I envy them for their carefree walking. An existence they don't even appreciate. The young woman in the dark gray coat at the bus stop probably has never thought about what her body does and that she just walks. However, I notice it. The walking of the people around me. And suddenly, I feel something like envy again. An almost shameful envy of people walking.

Amidst these people, I feel like an alien. I'm increasingly aware of how different our life has been since the illness began. In this society, we only lead a shadowy existence. Cut off from the outside world, I too spend most of my time in our apartment. Once I step outside, I see a different, new world. One that doesn't care about us. Occasionally our neighbor smiles at us. I smile back. Then she nods. Whatever these supposed conversations are meant to convey. They have nothing to do with genuine interest.

What do I expect? Even our longtime friends and acquaintances only sporadically inquire about Mia. Her friends contact her less and less. What value does such a friendship even hold, I wonder repeatedly. What are they all afraid of? Is it the fear of what they might encounter if they see Mia in this state? They wouldn't even have to come by. A small text message now and then, a brief call would suffice. A friendly inquiry. I almost find it audacious that they simply don't reach out. They would give us a sense of belonging if they only did. We wouldn't have to feel that we no longer belong to this society. What's so difficult about it, I wonder.

On the other hand, maybe I shouldn't be so harsh on them, I think then. They just don't know any better. No one knows what it's really like to be so excluded from life. From a life you want to be pulled back into. Even if only for a small moment. In a brief conversation, a little message. That would sometimes mean the world to us.

Even after Christmas, the days pass in a series of repetitive routines. Meanwhile, it's December 31st. For a few days, Mia has been experiencing pain in her left hip and knee. Yet, she doesn't complain, just mentions it.

Sometimes, when I look at her like this, I wonder how she copes with it all. How does she do it? In her vulnerability, she manages every day to maintain her own sense of dignity. It's as if she distances herself from the indignity of the moment and from what is happening to her. Despite being entirely dependent on others' help.

While washing her adult body. When I feed her. Change her diaper. Comb her hair. Or when dressing her.

She seems to let all these moments pass by without giving them too much attention. With a smile. With a joke or a deliberately chosen conversation about a beautiful memory from the past. One we can laugh about again.

And as for me? I consent to this game of pretending. Because it helps me too, to escape from what life is revealing to us, which should remain unnoticed. Our souls, after all, deserve sanctuary from the truths we might glimpse and feel if we dared. Only the clamorous moments can eclipse the quiet ones. For it's the quiet ones we shy away from hearing. It's in the hush that understanding seeps into our consciousness. Especially when we've paused fleetingly and are unprepared for what unfolds. Swiftly and unexpectedly. This realization. Of being trapped in a life not of our choosing. One we do not want in this form. And in those silent moments, fear of recognition lurks.

Hence, we drown out life with our loudest tones. With our resounding laughter over all that brings us happiness. Or once did. Now, I attempt to recapture that joy. With a medication we now await.

Yet my intuition repeatedly tells me I may have fixated too much on this medication. As if there were no other way out. I constantly cling to the thought that this treatment is the messiah bringing us salvation. Without the medication, nothing moves forward, a mantra persistently accompanying me.

However, I must free myself and seek my own alternatives. I've had enough of this waiting, of fearing someone might have a bad day and put their signature on the wrong document. Rejected instead of approved.

I need an outlet. Something to let me breathe. Something within my own discretion and in my hands. You were always so independent. Where has your fighting spirit gone? I ask myself. What have you become? A waiting, helpless mother? Just a beggar for a little dignity in her child's life? Transferring all responsibility to others because it's easier.

You could be searching for other solutions while waiting. For an escape route, in case the medication isn't approved. Especially since you were open to alternative healing approaches at the onset of the illness. Acupuncture, acupressure, homeopathy, cannabis—you left no stone unturned. You tried almost everything to make her feel better. Now, you just wait. Practically leaving her fate to the mood and goodwill of others.

Investigate! Read! Research! Find the escape route!, I admonish myself. Seek a way out of this misery.

"Because you always find the good in everything, Mom," as Mia often says.

Then finally find the good, I think in the evening on the couch. Tony, Mia, and I found a concert recording of our favorite singer on TV. Mia and I sing along, and I keep turning up the volume.

New Year's Eve on the couch, I think. And I don't care. We make the best of it. However, I care about my thoughts on the past year. Well, our happiness didn't last long, I think in the next moment. Just last year, Mia and I were in London, thinking we had left this illness behind us. We would have outsmarted it. Just a short episode in our existence, and we would have overtaken it in our sprint through life. With a quick glance back. Joyfully laughing because we had passed it. Almost unscathed. But the appearance was deceiving. It misled us for a brief moment.

Until our eyes were opened.

– Chapter 10 –

January 1, 2019

"You should say your goodbyes now," the doctor tells the woman.

She looks at him in disbelief. What does he mean? I should say my goodbyes. She squints, trying to read his next words from his face. Meanwhile, the loud beeping of the machines in the background becomes increasingly unbearable for her. Beep, beep, beep. Echoing in the same interval. In the same tone. Beep, beep, beep. It surprises her that her ears still register these sounds at all. The rushing in her head is so loud.

It's chilly in here, she thinks. And that smell of disinfectant. It briefly triggers a past memory before fading away. She still gazes at him. He must be in his early forties, she thinks, giving him a quick once-over. Short, somewhat stocky. But he's very confident in himself and his skills. Too confident. How could he say that? So casually. I should say my goodbyes.

"You'd better rest at home for a bit," he says hesitantly, avoiding her gaze. "Well, of course, I must inform you of the risks beforehand. There could be brain hemorrhages in this state. In the worst case scenario. From the lungs to the heart and then possibly to the brain. But we're not assuming that now. I just had to mention it."

She stares at him. Through him. Because his words only reach her in fragments. She has long shut herself off from what he's saying.

"In any case, we'll intervene if necessary. As I said, if there are brain hemorrhages. So far, only the lungs are affected. But for now, just go home. A cardiologist will be here soon to check the heart. You can come back tomorrow at any time. Even outside visiting hours," he concludes his explanation.

So, after those words, I'm supposed to go home, she thinks. With all that he has just seemingly nonchalantly recounted to me. As if he were in a lecture, explaining to his students the progression of an escalating illness. A patient's story ending tragically. For him, it seems to be just a story, she thinks in the next moment.

Now I'm supposed to leave with this knowledge, she concludes. Knowing that tomorrow I could encounter a completely different person here. One who is no longer responsive. Who doesn't recognize me. Doesn't even see me. Because she's no longer conscious. Or even worse…

Her heart starts pounding wildly. Suddenly, she feels like she could faint here and now at the thought of the worst scenario. She wants to scream. Loudly. To scream out her pain as loudly as possible. She trembles all over.

What should she say? A simple "See you tomorrow…"? Or should she express once again all that you say when it could be the last words to your most beloved. Your child. What should I say, she wants to scream. What should I do? Her body seems paralyzed by this question. She feels panic rising within her. In her desperation, she just wants to close her eyes and fall asleep. Please let me fall asleep! Let it finally be over. I can't take it anymore.

How can she bear this? The loss of her own child. Nothing matters anymore. She just wants to fall asleep and never wake up. In this glassed room of the intensive care unit. She wants to lie down next to her daughter. Among all the tubes and wires. To hold her close and breathe in her scent. That's where she wants to stay. The woman.

This woman is me.

By now, Tony and I are in the car on our way home. After bidding a heartfelt farewell to Mia in anticipation of seeing her again tomorrow, I was able to leave the hospital. Of course, she joked about the whole ordeal. That's typical Mia, after all. She lay there, connected to all those machines, with a confident smile as if nothing had happened. I couldn't detect any fear in her eyes. Not a single spark.

As for me, the fear threatens to tear me apart from within. Is she misinterpreting the situation, and that's why she remains so relaxed? I, however, remain vigilant, I think, while staring out the passenger window at the empty streets. I won't relax for a moment or just watch things unfold. Feeling like a hunted animal, I remain alert. It's this constant feeling of fear, as if danger lurks everywhere. A danger that renders me powerless. How could this happen? I ask myself. Should I have recognized the signs earlier? Why didn't you pay better attention? Why did it have to go so far? To a pulmonary embolism.

She was fine on New Year's Eve. It was only on the morning of January 1st, during our exercises on the couch, that I noticed her left leg was so difficult to lift. Suddenly, it looked swollen. Was it because she had been lying down constantly, I wondered. We need to elevate it, I thought. But by noon, nothing had changed. It was still swollen. From the ankle up to the hip.

Either we sit around here and wait for it to subside, or we take action, I thought. That doesn't look normal somehow. Tony agreed that we should get it checked out. Mia, however, seemed alarmed by the fact that we were going to the hospital on January 1st. The anxiety about possibly having to stay in the clinic again was written all over her face.

In the emergency room, the diagnosis was quickly made after an extensive ultrasound. Deep vein thrombosis in two places.

"How can that be? She was fine just yesterday," I asked the doctor, disbelief evident in my voice.

"Be glad you caught it at all," he replied. "Sometimes, these things seem to happen overnight and can have far-reaching consequences if unnoticed."

After that, everything happened quickly. Doctor Harper was consulted over the phone to determine what needed attention from a neurological standpoint. For now, it appeared there were no neurological concerns to address alongside the thrombosis, as indicated by the internist's nod.

"Okay. Very active MS," he whispered almost to himself. "Alright, let's take things one step at a time and focus on the thrombosis first."

That's right, I thought. Because the medication is still pending approval. Don't they understand that this is urgent? The board must say yes now, raced through my mind. They can't be that heartless. Especially now that it's gotten to this point.

Four days later, around eleven, Tony and I arrived at the internal medicine ward to visit Mia, when a scene unfolded in the hallway that I now ponder on as we drive back. It was a kind of déjà vu, in a way, because this scene felt oddly familiar. And it still sends shivers down my spine.

From a distance, I could see two nurses rushing into Mia's room with a large oxygen tank. There was a palpable sense of urgency all around. One nurse was pushing a cart with the tank, while the other held the door open to the room.

"What's going on?" I asked, and hurried down the hallway to Mia's room.

One of the nurses quickly explained that Mia had complained of difficulty breathing during breakfast. Something was off with her oxygen saturation. So she needed oxygen immediately.

Mia just lay there. Her right index finger connected to a device that apparently measured oxygen saturation. It must be a hundred, I thought, as I stared at the device for a moment. Why is it so low? Why is this happening now?

Hardly had I exchanged a few words with Mia while crouching beside her, stroking her head, when one of the nurses stood beside me.

"We need to go to the CT scan immediately," she explained kindly but with an undertone of impatience. "We're just waiting for the internist from Ward Seven, who accompanies Mia. That's how it is in emergencies. We can't take her down alone in this condition. A doctor must be present," she finished the sentence.

Meanwhile, the doctor she mentioned emerged from the nearby elevator. His haste was evident as he made his way toward us. He appeared rather young, I thought briefly, and in no time, I found myself, along with Tony, hurrying down the long hospital corridors alongside him. A nurse, accompanied by the doctor, wheeled Mia in her hospital bed. An obvious surge of adrenaline propelled me to keep pace with the doctor's long and brisk strides, as if I were running a marathon.

About thirty minutes later, Tony and I were back in the hallway of the internal medicine ward, waiting for the CT results.

"Could you please come with me for a moment?" the young doctor asked me, gesturing for me to join him in the nurses' station.

"Mia has a pulmonary embolism. Despite the blood-thinning medication, the blood clots in her left leg have traveled to her lungs," he explained, giving me a scrutinizing look.

"Okay," I responded cautiously. I immediately grasped the gravity of the situation. A pulmonary embolism can be fatal. I had seen too many reports on TV of both celebrities and ordinary people who had died unexpectedly from a pulmonary embolism, often going unnoticed.

"How… how bad is it?" I asked, hoping for a reassuring answer, something like: "It doesn't look so bad. Just a tiny spot. It'll be over by tomorrow."

"Well, I have to be honest with you. If we differentiate between a milder and a more severe embolism, then this is a more severe one," he replied, looking at me.

Suddenly, one of the nurses stood beside me and offered me a seat on a small swivel chair in the tiny nurses' station.

"Come, have a seat. Here, take this for now. For calming down."

I swallowed a pill, which must have been a sedative. Obviously, my shock and rising panic were evident. Why was the nurse looking at me with such concern?

Then everything happened in a blur. Mia was transferred to the intensive care unit.

"Mom," she whispered to me once we arrived there. "They want me to take off the ring. My ring from London." She looked at me, tears welling in her eyes, choking me up.

"It's just because of all these machines. Tomorrow I'll bring it back to you, sweetie. Don't worry," I replied, trying to sound casual.

Her ring, I think now in the car, as Tony and I drive home through the dark streets of the city. The silver ring with the turquoise stone I bought for her in London. On Portobello Road. Back when everything seemed alright with the world.

When I get home, I head straight for our bathroom. Even though I hate taking these pills, I need something to calm me down now. How else am I supposed to make it through the rest of the evening? Especially since Mia is scheduled for an examination by a cardiologist in the intensive care unit today. Maybe he's already there, I think, as my heart pounds wildly in my chest. "From the lungs to the heart, then to the brain," the internist in the intensive care unit said earlier.

I refuse to accept that, I think in the next moment. Something like that shouldn't happen. I look into the bathroom mirror. Look into my own eyes. And for the first time in my life, I wonder what it feels like to go crazy. When something in you goes crazy. Do you notice it? Is it like suddenly crossing a border? As if you're stepping from solid ground into water. But in between, there's something. A kind of door threshold that you touch with your foot.

Is it like that? Or is the boundary so blurred that you don't notice it and just transition from one state to another? The mind floating. From sane to insane. Just feeling the unbearable in the here and now. And in the next moment, being in a different reality.

I quickly swallow the calming pill and wash my face with cold water. No, this won't happen to you, I warn my reflection. You stay here. Here in this bathroom. In your reality. The one where Mia is waiting for all of this to pass. And you're there for her. You don't have time to go crazy. It's a waste of time.

My gaze falls on her hairbrush. Her beautiful, long, golden-brown hair, I think, and tears of despair run down my face. And then there's … her perfume. I'm afraid to smell it. The associated memory of her once carefree life is too painful. When she could leave the house in the morning to go to university. Back then.

What has she done to you? I want to scream. Take me instead and spare her! Until now, you've been my rock, my anchor, my unwavering belief that all things eventually fall into place. No matter what happens. Why have You turned against me, disregarding and betraying my trust? Haven't I shown you abundantly that I don't turn away from you even in difficult times? Even in moments when I had no explanation for any of this. Haven't I always defended you, held up my shield to protect you, and remained loyal to you? Always waiting trustingly for your higher meaning in all of this. In a way, for the resolution.

The moral of the story.

And now? Now I'm supposed to give up my only child? Which of my sins could possibly weigh so heavily? No! I can't do this anymore! I'm not ready to bear this burden. Take me. I won't give her up!

What in the world is happening with Doctor Harper? I wonder impatiently the next morning. Especially now, with Mia in intensive care, he could expedite this approval process.

The thought of him makes me increasingly angry. And I increasingly wonder if he's indifferent to Mia's fate. These days I haven't had a chance to speak with him. Neither by phone nor in person. He seems only accessible for his colleagues. The disappointment over this apparent indifference further frays my already weak nerves.

Despite the good news from the clinic last night about the cardiological examination, I'm still on edge. What comes next, I wonder. The doctors want to keep Mia in intensive care for another night. For observation. Then she could be transferred to neurology. Because of the underlying condition.

Underlying condition, I muse. As if that isn't enough already. At the onset of the illness, I couldn't have imagined that MS could lead to so many additional conditions. Not even remotely. Vision loss, paralysis in arms and legs. That was already clear to me. But the whole package. No, I hadn't envisioned it escalating like this.

What will become of her? I think to myself early in the afternoon, while sitting at my desk. Five days have passed since Mia was admitted to the hospital on New Year's Day. It's hardly possible to concentrate on my translations anymore. The paperwork for accounting also remains untouched in the top desk drawer, waiting to be sorted, signed, and stamped.

"I just can't," I whisper to myself, glancing at the numerous unanswered emails in my inbox. Translation requests from clients I've been working with for years. I can't just leave them hanging, but I can't muster the strength somehow.

That's why I decide to offer them later delivery dates. It's the only way I can manage it. How am I supposed to focus on their financial statements, descriptions of medical devices, or any presentations? And still provide the usual quality.

On the other hand, my company must keep running. Even though I wish life would just pause here and wait for me. Until everything gets better. Until I can live and work again. Until

I'm able to redirect my thoughts to something other than the ordeal we're currently facing. This never-ending state of shock.

Among the emails, there are inquiries from new clients as well. I indifferently forward them to the rival companies. Because I don't care who profits from it. Who cashes in on all those big translation deals. Who reels in new clients. I'm only concerned about how I'll get through the next day, to witness my child getting better.

Suddenly I remember dreaming of Mia in a wheelchair last night. Tears of shame burn in my eyes at the thought of this dream as I stare at the laptop screen. You can't dream something like that! It's just not right. Like that, you're betraying her in a way. Not even in your subconscious should this thought be present, I remind myself more insistently, shaking my head. As if I could shake the thoughts from my mind.

Then my eyes land on Mia's childhood photos on the wall above my desk. Especially on one where she's about three years old. A summer on the island. Mia stands on a path lined with pine trees and vacation homes. We're on our way to her friend Maya's. For playtime. She smiles at me in her mischievous way. In her blue T-shirt and short white pants. How carefree life was back then. How easily happiness seemed within reach. Just an ordinary stroll. The prospect of a fun afternoon with her friend Maya. Playing tag, dressing and undressing dolls, chasing the kittens in the garden, eating a pack of peanut flips together. Accidentally spilling half the contents of the pack on the floor and picking them up again.

Just a typical afternoon in the life of a three-year-old, I think now, and it chokes me up.

Today, I know how life actually unfolds. Unpredictable. Above all, it's exactly that. Unpredictable. The thought of it terrifies me when I think about Mia's later life. Who will take care of her one day when I'm no longer here? Who will care for her in her old age? Never before have I pondered this question. Until now, I haven't dared to think about such a distant future.

One where I can't make a difference anymore. A topic like 'care' has never crossed my mind before. Briefly, an imaginary scene from a nursing home flashes in my mind.

"No!" I banish it loudly from my thoughts and turn my gaze away from Mia's photo.

Yet, I must confront this question. Somehow, I must provide for her. Care is expensive. That's well known. Very expensive. With these thoughts, panic rises within me. How can I possibly ensure her financial security into old age? How much will that even be? I have to calculate that. All these thoughts are racing through my mind. I need to know how much she needs to be taken care of.

In theory, children should take care of their parents, I think in the next moment, staring into space. But… will she even have children? In this condition? Can she meet a man like that? One who accepts her as she is.

Women and men can split up, I then think. Children stay. At best, they turn out well, and you can rely on them. She should have at least one. One with whom she shares a bond as close as hers and mine. Like her and me. Mia and Mommy, I think then, recalling all the pictures she painted for me in kindergarten. On each picture, she had written "Mia and Mommy" and had drawn a heart next to it.

"I wish this for you," I whisper, tears streaming down. A love that lasts forever. The love between mother and child. One you can lean on.

Truly lean on.

The days drag on without me taking notice. Each day overlays the other like a template, with no variation. Gray and soundless. It gets harder for me each morning to get up and ready for the day. As soon as I open my eyes, I realize the life I'm living. Not the life I once imagined. Especially not for Mia.

To make matters worse, I'm haunted by nightmares while I sleep, where I'm carrying her because she can't walk. Or I'm pushing her around in a wheelchair. Honestly, I don't know which is worse. The fact that she doesn't walk in my dreams anymore. Or the realization that this could be a product of what I actually believe. Consciously, I believe she'll walk again. But what do I truly believe, I wonder in those moments. When I have dreams like these. Why don't you dream what you believe in? I ask myself. About the walking Mia. The one who can do everything again. The young, lively student living carefree. That's who we want to get back to. Then why do you dream about wheelchairs, about carrying and pushing?

It's only for her that you muster the strength every day to be part of this life, to strive towards another one. And that must be reinforced in my thoughts, I remind myself each time. Mia is healthy. Mia is perfectly healthy. That's my new daily positive affirmation. I repeat it over and over again in my thoughts. Because that's the only way forward. This thought should solidify to the point where it can and must only be the truth. And our reality.

Meanwhile, Mia has been transferred from the intensive care unit to cardiology and then to neurology. The interim stop was because there were no available beds in the neurology ward. Of course, it's not particularly pleasant for patients. Constantly moving back and forth. One moment in this room with these bed neighbors and nurses. Then a completely different environment. Familiarity doesn't come quickly, and in recent days, Mia's impatience to be transferred to neurology could be felt. At least she knows the nurses, the rooms, the routines here.

So now she's back in Room 7 in neurology. Immobile, with a bladder catheter and her left leg elevated in a compression bandage. And yet, despite it all, brave and seemingly cheerful.

On the neurology ward itself, however, there's been a strange atmosphere lately when Tony and I arrive. They respond irritably and dismissively to my inquiries about where Doctor

Harper is and what the treatment plan is. That's not like them at all, I think.

Maybe it's because Tony and I make the most of visiting hours from the first minute to the last. We come and go right on the dot. Perhaps we're disrupting their routine? Perhaps the nurses prefer some peace and quiet. No annoying questions from family members.

Even my overly friendly tone seems to fall flat with them. Especially when it comes to questions about therapy. Nobody wants to talk about it here, my gut tells me. Even doctors I stop in passing wave me off, saying they have no information. I have to ask Doctor Harper, they say. In moments like these, I feel like nobody knows what to do. They'd rather stay silent and ignore me.

Except for one young doctor who lets slip a single sentence about the B-cell therapy question one afternoon.

"Well, all I know is that Doctor Harper presents to the board every week. They drag it out, and he's not happy about it. That's all I can tell you," she finishes, those few but precious sentences hanging in the air.

He's trying, I think. Mia matters to him. She's not just another patient, someone he doesn't give a second thought to. And that gives me hope again. But as quickly as hope flares up in me, it vanishes, replaced by doubt.

I want to speak with someone on the ward about Mia's ongoing treatment here in neurology and when she'll be discharged. Can anything be done until she gets the medication? Besides treating the thrombosis and embolism with blood thinners. Especially since nobody tells me how it happened. Was it the prolonged lying? Or perhaps, as I read online, the excessive doses of corticosteroids last summer and fall. She received an abundance of those. Out of sheer desperation from the doctors? To avoid standing by idly. Or to avoid witnessing a young woman slowly but surely become a long-term nursing care case?

I want to know what happens next for her here. I certainly won't spend my days waiting for her to be discharged from the hospital—with no answers and no therapy. I want answers. And a treatment plan.

That's why, during a typical afternoon visit to the hospital, I seize the opportunity to talk to someone. It's been about a week since Mia arrived in neurology, and I can't and won't be put off any longer.

Tony stays in the patient's room with Mia while I linger in the hallway, hoping to find an receptive nurse. Spotting a ward nurse I recognize, I approach her. She's the one who seemed too prim to bathe Mia, I briefly recall, but I quickly push that thought aside. I want to approach her with a positive attitude. If that's even possible here—amidst the smell of urine bags and the constant calls from patients' rooms.

When I speak to her, she seems eager to keep walking, but I stop her.

She's about Mia's age. I know because Mia follows her on social media. Medium height. Slim figure, yet somehow provocative as she struts from room to room. Dark, shoulder-length hair. Always perfectly groomed. Makeup, powder, blush, red-painted lips. And long, black, artificial lashes. Lashes that somehow irk me here on the ward. I can't help feeling that every time I see those lashes, this nurse doesn't know where she is. And I almost feel provoked by this exaggeration.

Mia is about the same age. Probably that's why. Seeing the ward nurse all dolled up hurts. Because my daughter lies on this ward in diapers with a bladder catheter. It makes me involuntarily angry, and honestly … honestly, it makes me want to peel off her fake lashes. But that's nonsense, of course, I think as I stand in the hallway with her.

"Nurse, I have a question. Do you know how Mia will be treated in the coming days? I mean, besides the blood thinners. What about her MS? She can't stay like this."

"Unfortunately, I don't know," she replies, turning to leave.

"But someone must know something. I haven't seen the head nurse for days. No one gives Mia any information during rounds. Do you at least know how long she has to stay here?"

"No, you'll have to ask the doctor. I really don't know," she replies.

I take a step back to escape the cloud of her overpowering perfume. Still, I force myself to keep smiling as we talk. After all, she's not to blame for the lack of information she's trying to explain to me.

Which makes her sudden remark, in a tone that sounds accusing to my ears, all the more surprising.

"But, what I wanted to ask. We noticed that Mia has a pressure sore at her tailbone. About two, three centimeters in size. Didn't you see that?" She looks at me through her meticulously made-up eyes, and suddenly, I feel like I'm standing in front of a high school teacher.

"No, I didn't see it," I reply in my most convincing tone. "Otherwise, I would have definitely taken care of it. Or what do you think?" I meet her gaze.

"Not even while changing her diaper?"

"Listen, Nurse!" I briefly glance at her name tag on the collar of her nursing uniform: "Nurse Helen. If I had seen that, it wouldn't be there now. Because I certainly would have treated that wound," I explain, trying to maintain my calm demeanor. "But you've taken care of it now," I add, smiling at her once more. With that, the conversation concludes for me at this moment, and I head back to Room 7, where Mia and Tony are waiting for me.

Actually, I should have explained to her how I missed it. That's what she expected. She expected me to justify myself. I should have told her how I turn Mia when washing and changing diapers. That I'm not an experienced nurse. Especially considering I handle everything alone, using a bed or couch not designed for these tasks. Doing it the way that's best for Mia in that moment. So that it takes up as little space as possible in our everyday life. So we can overlook it. Don't have to make a big fuss about it.

But before stepping into Mia's room, I remind myself: No one has the right to blame me for anything here. And certainly not that nurse with her false lashes. Who does she think she is?!

Friday, January 18, 2019

Nearly three weeks after her admission, Mia is discharged from the hospital on a Friday morning. Still in her previous condition. Immobile. In diapers. Only this time, there is also a thrombosis stocking on her left leg. As if the ordeal of the MS symptoms weren't enough.

So, here we are again, I think as we arrive home. The same routine all over again. Tony carries her up the stairs to the apartment from the car and lays her on the couch. Now we have to make sure her left leg is elevated, also. And the thrombosis stocking can't even be taken off at night.

"Just during bathing," the head nurse explained to me early this morning before handing over the discharge papers.

Okay, I thought, we can handle that.

But what about Mia, I wonder now. How much longer can she endure this? With no prospect of quick improvement. I'm just the small bandage on the wound here. The helping hand. The comforting word. Yet, she must endure it alone. Trapped inside her own body.

Once again, she has shown how to weather such a setback. At least outwardly. Most of the time, she's cheerful. But when I look at her when she's unaware, she seems introspective. Thoughtful. It must look very different inside, I think again and again. I'm aware of the thoughts that plague her. And then there's this powerlessness. The utter dependence on others. Even if it's her own mother. That provides little comfort in light of the actual situation.

At least she's glad to be home. Able to sleep in her own bed, she says. Or at least in our parents' bed. In her favorite bedding, which smells of familiarity and comfort. Yet nothing is the same as it once was. We don't need to say it aloud. The three of us know it and stay silent. That cozy feeling only scratches the surface because once we look deeper within ourselves, everything is different. No fragrant bedding, no shared laughter, no familiar TV nights can mask it. Perhaps for a moment. But this moment never lasts long.

In my mind, the illness is always present. I constantly ponder its course and how I can change it.

Especially over the past few nights, while Mia was still in neurology. Tony slept peacefully beside me. Just when I should have been doing the same, the same carousel of doubts and hopes always began spinning. About why things turned out this way and what solution I can and must find. And sometimes, terrible thoughts flashed through my mind, which I quickly banished. You have to think pragmatically, I reminded myself.

I didn't see a treatment plan at the clinic, not by any means, so I redirected my thoughts and looked up at the bedroom ceiling.

Basically, early on in Mia's current hospital stay, I realized that the doctors were uncertain about how to proceed with her treatment. In any case, she can't receive corticosteroids anymore. They undoubtedly contributed to the pulmonary embolism. While this fact hasn't been officially confirmed. It's not mentioned in any preliminary report. Likely because it would be an admission of their limited treatment options. At least, it's limited without this medication we're waiting for.

Well, that medication. OC. What about this holy grail of MS? How effective is it really, I constantly wondered in these nights. I mean, we're waiting for something that's supposed to get Mia back on her feet. From a condition that seems beyond hopeless. Do the ingredients in this medication even have the potential to lead to a full recovery? In the end, we might be waiting and relying on something that doesn't bring us the desired success.

Because what we want is a mostly complete recovery. Walking, eating independently, bathing, using the bathroom. And leaving the house alone, going for a coffee with friends, attending the theater, navigating the subway independently. Returning to studies and work. Including longer walks, flights of stairs, and everything a healthy person takes for granted.

Can OC make that happen?

After days of internet research, my layman's conclusion is this: it seems somewhat possible, but not impossible.

Some scientific studies, for example, suggest that one can remain more or less relapse-free for at least two years after the second dose of medication. That would mean Mia's condition would stay the same. Without significant deterioration.

But then I wonder: Can it get any worse, as I read these facts in a medical study. How can it get any worse than bad? That would mean her condition remains as it is now. And ironically, that fact brings me some comfort. At least then she won't have to endure relapses anymore. Even if everything stays the same. I'll count it as a positive, I think, going through the list in my head.

As for the effect on the progression of disability, the study further states that the time until patients need a wheelchair is delayed by about seven years.

And what does that mean for those patients who are already in a wheelchair or can't even sit at all? What does that mean? What is to be delayed when we've already arrived there long ago? Delay simply means the disease doesn't progress as quickly, I conclude. However, there's no mention of regaining lost functions. So it's progressing slower.

But does it also regress? The clinic remains silent on the effects of OC. Probably to prevent us from building up too much hope about the medication, I've already concluded. That's why

I must find out alone what we can expect. And what we can't. But how do you interpret these data individually? Tailored to us, so to speak.

As I continue reading, I come across the familiar disability scale. Values from 0 to 10 are listed. Where 0 means no disability and 10, well, what we're experiencing right now. I don't want to admit it. But it's probably true. It's a 10.

How do we go from 10 to 0 now, I wonder. That would be the ideal scenario, of course. Would you have thought last year that you would be happy about a 1 on this scale, I wonder in the next moment. A 5 would be a milestone. The first supported steps would already rank as a 7 or 8 on my own scale. By now, it's difficult to imagine what it would be like if she were back on her feet, even taking a step or two. It all seems so far away. In a distant past.

I read and read. Studies upon studies. Then the package insert of the medication, which can be viewed on the drug manufacturer's website. I read for hours, even days.

Of course, also about the side effects. I can't ignore those. But then I wonder, how significant are they on my scale of benefits and harms. Almost insignificant. This whole illness is one big side effect. It's there beside us, hindering us from living our lives. As if it's walking alongside us. Uninvited and relentless.

After all the data and facts, to me, it means this medication must be able to do something. Delaying means it's working. Effect means change, I contemplate. And change, in our case, means improvement. Because the path leads only forward now. There's simply no room to move backward. There's no space between the back and the wall.

That's why this medication is so important for Mia.

On the same day, around half past six in the evening, my phone rings. I'm in the bedroom, remaking the bed. Mia and Tony are in the living room. I hear them laughing loudly. They're talking about some nonsense they find worth discussing. Because it's fun. And because Mia is finally back home.

I smile, glancing at my phone display before answering the call. I don't recognize this number. Probably a client, I think.

The conversation is brief. But it will undoubtedly sear into my memory. It's Doctor Harper. I recognize that tone in his voice before he even finishes his first sentence.

"Is Mia nearby?" he asks, and in that moment, a world collapses for me. Because I know what that question means.

It's over. All the conjectures and plans I had about an approval, the anticipation, and all my hopes crumble to dust in that instant.

Rejected. Only that one word echoes in my head. Rejected.

He mentions a donation in the last sentence before we say goodbye. However, I barely register this as a last resort.

It's over. The board said no. Just like that.

After hanging up, I briefly consider going to the hospital. To tell them what I think about the rejection. To vent all my frustration and anger that has built up inside me.

Instead, I go to the bathroom, sit on the edge of the bathtub, and cry. I cry tears of injustice. Tears of despair and hopelessness that this one message makes me acutely aware of. Because how are we supposed to go on now? When I'm honest with myself, I realize now I had already counted on them approving the medication. That thought had solidified in my mind. Now, my entire framework of thought has evaporated. Like a pink cloud of dust. Leaving behind not even a hint of hope. Because until now, I had at least lived with that hope.

How could I have been so naive? I wonder, shaking my head in disbelief. Why were you so foolish to place your trust in that? You wasted valuable time when you could have been looking for other solutions. How foolish to believe the board would read your letter and your words would evoke some compassion in the members. Compassion. What do they know about that, I whisper, choking back bitter tears of injustice. I feel disregarded. That's it. Disregarded and abandoned. So they prefer to do nothing and leave Mia to her fate. Just like that.

A few minutes later, I change and make up an excuse to leave the apartment. "Need to grab something quick at the pharmacy," I call out to Mia and Tony from the hallway before shutting the door behind me. "It's almost seven o'clock, and the pharmacy's about to close."

Stepping outside, I enter the darkness of this cold January evening. My body shivers. But it's not from the cold seeping into me. Rather, it's the certainty that I can now let my thoughts roam freely that frightens me.

Pausing briefly outside our building, I try to calm my racing heart. Four seconds inhale, four hold, four exhale. A gentle breeze brushes my face, and I close my eyes for a moment.

As I start walking, I realize how safe I feel out here in the darkness. Because on the street, no one sees me. In the silence, without the gaze of the few passing pedestrians, I can delve into my thoughts as I make my way to the pharmacy, just two streets away. I don't have to answer any questions or owe anyone an explanation for the tears streaming down my face. Out here in the dark, there's only me. Me and my thoughts.

How could all this happen, I wonder. Why did the board say no? I was almost certain things would turn out for the best. How can Mia go on like this? And most importantly, how can I help her? Something needs to be done. But not someday, but right now. She's been in this state for too long. Her body, all those nerve cells… how will they recover if we wait too long?

I need to find a solution fast, it comes to my mind, and this urgency stabs at my heart once more. Everything needs to happen fast. So she can be like she was before. Time is slipping away from us. My gut tells me we can't wait forever for treatment.

I wish I could freeze time, so life wouldn't move on without us. Plant a stake in the ground and anchor time to it. Make it hold, waiting for us until we're ready to dive back into life. Everything should stay as it is until Mia is back on her feet, so we can step into the world we once knew. When that moment arrives. When Mia has recovered. When she… walks again, I think, and it almost sounds strange in my mind to even think about it.

When she walks again. Sometimes, I can barely conjure up that feeling of walking beside her. On walks, during errands. Laughing, joking, always full of plans for what's next or in conversation about how the day went. What happened at university today? How was work? Where are you going later?

The memory of those carefree days briefly brings me joy. But in the next moment, it plunges me into unspeakable pain.

So I rigorously attempt to banish every dark thought to the farthest corners of my mind. However, at least for the short walk to the pharmacy, I allow myself to imagine it, I think to myself. Just that brief stretch, I try to envision how it will be when she walks again. And dances. And jumps. And runs.

And lives her life.

Sunday, January 19, 2019

I never thought this illness, with all its accompanying surprises, could catch me off guard again. But it can. And it proves it to me early on Saturday morning. Just one day after Mia's discharge from the hospital and the rejection from the medical board.

Right after breakfast, while I'm changing Mia's diaper on the couch, she complains of abdominal pain. She says it hurts when I turn her onto her side, and suddenly, I notice how unusually swollen her abdomen appears. This has only happened before when she hasn't emptied her bowels for more than two days. But this time, it looks different. And not in a good way, I think, deciding in that moment not to wait any longer.

"Tony," I call out toward the kitchen. "We need to get to the emergency room right away. Something's not right with Mia's abdomen."

After two hours of waiting among the many patients in the crowded emergency room, it turns out Mia's bladder is dangerously full. At least, that's how the urologist puts it. The ultrasound reveals a lot of dark fluid, which turns out to be urine that Mia apparently hasn't been able to pass since yesterday. So, they insert a bladder catheter to empty her bladder.

The urologist asks Mia if she felt anything unusual.

No, she didn't. It only hurt a bit this morning.

"That's unusual," the doctor remarks, given the amount of fluid. "Normally, it's unbearable and causes intense pain."

"Well, that's probably because I don't feel much anyway," Mia responds. "I have numbness almost all over my body. Almost everything is numb."

"That's often the case with MS," the urologist explains, and then instructs the nurse in the treatment room to insert an indwelling catheter. Mia will need it for a while, until her bladder functions normally again.

Shortly after, when I ask, the nurse quickly demonstrates how to change the urine bag at home—and that's it for now.

"You'll get the urine bags prescribed by your general practitioner. Change the bag when it's full. Follow-up in two weeks," she says.

And then we're discharged home.

As if our situation isn't enough, Mia now needs an indwelling catheter on top of everything else.

Wonderful, I think as I sit in the car a little later. Now she needs a bag too.

Mia is lying on the back seat, Tony and I sit in the front. We're all silent. Even Mia, who usually has a joke ready for any situation, seems to want peace and quiet on the way home.

I gaze out of the passenger window, trying to mentally prepare for how to change the bag at home. Because I want to be ready in an hour or two. I couldn't think clearly in the emergency room anyway.

Well, I think, I use disposable latex gloves every day for changing diapers. My fingernails are short, so they won't tear the gloves. But does anything else need to be sterile when I remove the urine bag from the tube? I wonder the next moment, furrowing my brow. No one mentioned that. And how do I stop the urine in the tube itself when there's no bag attached? The nurse seemed to just hold it up to prevent any leakage until she unscrewed one bag and attached the next. These are the little details nobody explains, I think to myself

Okay, I think to myself, trying to muster some courage. We've managed everything so far. We'll manage this too. We won't keep that thing for long anyway. I'll make sure of that.

Yes, I'll make sure of it, I think later in the evening, staring into the bathroom mirror. Sometimes, I hardly recognize myself as I look in the mirror. Not long ago, I'd never leave the house without makeup or my contact lenses. Now I quickly cover my dark circles for a hospital visit at most, and put on my glasses. Even the gray streaks in my hair don't faze me anymore.

But I can't erase the traces of my tears, I think bitterly. The skin around my eyes is reddened from countless silent tears. I've splashed my face with ice-cold water several times already, quietly blowing my nose. Then, I turn on the faucet in the bathtub repeatedly, creating the illusion that I'm cleaning it in the living room.

Since we left the emergency room this morning, I've been crying silently here several times, the only place where nobody can see me.

My thoughts have been consumed by what I can do to help Mia since Friday's rejection. Today's bladder incident only reaffirmed that things can't continue like this. And it fills me with anger and sadness. So I cry. I cry to release the constant pressure. To avoid screaming. To remain patient when Mia needs something.

When I have to redo her hair for the hundredth time because the ponytail hurts when she lies down.

When the diaper isn't positioned right and causes discomfort.

When I make a mess while feeding her.

When the water in the turquoise plastic tub isn't warm enough to bathe her.

And then a customer calls. Over something trivial. A silly word he wants changed in a translation. A delivery time he wants moved up. Something that could throw me off balance.

That's why I cry in the bathroom. So I don't take out all this pent-up frustration on Mia. Because she doesn't deserve that. She needs a loving mother. One who knows how to radiate patience and optimism, no matter the circumstance.

That's why I need these moments alone in the bathroom. Moments before I leave the bathroom and quickly walk through the living room to the adjacent kitchen. Because Mia might notice the tears I've shed.

Then I turn up the music on the radio and cheerfully announce to Mia that our favorite song might be coming on soon. I hum along to the songs on the radio to relax. Just for one or two minutes. Only until I feel better. Until I'm ready to go back to the living room and be a happy mother for Mia. The mother she deserves. The mother she needs right now.

– Chapter 11 –

Sunday, January 20, 2019

As much as I've searched for an explanation in the past two days for why the medication treatment was rejected, I decide I have to come to terms with it for now. It was probably a matter of budget. The first medication didn't help Mia and was already very expensive. Why would the second one work better, and why would they spend money on the same patient again? A patient whose condition seems hopeless in the eyes of the medical board. They'd rather give the funds to someone for whom it's still considered worthwhile. That must be how the board justified their decision, I keep thinking.

But ultimately, what's the point here? It's about getting my daughter Mia back on her feet and living a normal life. There's no use pondering how the board members could be so heartless. And why.

I have to take action. Step one is securing the medication. I've decided I need to find a way through donations. And step two is what I've been researching for weeks and can tackle immediately: utilizing our body's self-healing abilities and understanding what positive thinking and the right mindset can truly achieve.

Whether it's just the ramblings of some enlightened positive thinkers who spend their days painting rosy pictures. Or if it's somehow demonstrable and possibly scientifically grounded.

That's why I'm starting from scratch. What about our brain, our command center, and our thoughts?

First, I recall that movements are largely controlled by the brain. So, from where inflammation occurs in Multiple Sclerosis. For the motor commands sent by the brain to be carried out, they must reach the muscles. So the pathway goes from the brain through the command to the muscles. Specialized nerve pathways in the spinal cord act as intermediaries between command and muscle, like highways.

Now, I wonder, what if these nerve pathways stop functioning, and how does that relate to positive thinking?

And I continue reading.

The human brain is evolutionarily predisposed to negative thoughts. When our ancestors woke up in the morning, they weren't thinking, 'What a wonderful day, I'll just relax today.'

Instead, they thought, 'I haven't eaten in two days. I need some meat. Let's hunt!'

Instincts back then mainly promoted thoughts focused on survival. And that included danger. Danger was everywhere. Mammoth, neighbor, rival tribe, food thief. Looking at the lives of our ancient ancestors from today's perspective, their daily routine seems to have been primarily shaped by negative thoughts.

It appears that over the course of evolution, we've become accustomed to this.

So what exactly do these negative thoughts trigger in our bodies? After all, everyone knows the feeling when a single, even fleeting thought unleashes a flood of symptoms within our own body. Stomach pains, a pang in the heart, headaches, or just a general sense of discomfort. Thoughts have the power to ignite a specific feeling within us, along with an associated physical symptom. Whether it's a pleasant thought with a comforting feeling or a negative thought that brings about discomfort in turn.

So far, so good. Up to this point, no scientific evidence is needed to convince me. I'm well aware of this cause-and-effect relationship. Just thinking about unpaid bills gives me a stomachache. Once the bills are paid, I feel relief just by thinking about it.

If our thoughts can trigger a certain feeling within us, I ask myself further, what processes set these feelings in motion within our bodies? And how does this relate to our nerves?

A plausible answer seems to be the chemical processes triggered by thoughts and emotions in our body. Because thoughts have a specific influence on our bodily processes. As well as on the hormonal system, the cardiovascular system, and our immune system.

Each thought releases certain biochemical messengers that affect our metabolism. These messengers, in turn, have a direct impact on our well-being and our body cells. I read further that a certain protein synthesis constantly takes place in our cells. Since our nerve cells continuously require new proteins, this consequently has a positive effect on our nerve cells.

So with every thought and change in emotion, the tone of our nervous system changes. Such changes are even visible in our brain. Using modern imaging techniques like MRI, precise brainwave recordings in real time remarkably illustrate how our thoughts affect our brain.

And all this happens with both positive and negative thoughts. Sometimes helpful, sometimes harmful.

With about seventy thousand thoughts a person thinks daily, you thus have the choice of which type of messengers you would prefer. Because each of these myriad thoughts carries the potential to make us feel good or bad. It's just a matter of which direction we steer our thoughts.

Everyone knows the question: Is the glass half full or half empty? What sounds like a worn-out cliché, for the quintessential positive thinker actually seems to be an opportunity to determine where the journey goes. Into a life filled with positive thoughts that release good messengers in our body, causing pleasant feelings that positively influence our cells. Or a journey in the other direction.

And we have this choice every day. Over and over again. Why does it still seem so odd to some people to think positively, I wonder. Positive thinkers are often considered peculiar, unrealistic, or naive. Negative thinking, on the other hand, is seen as realistic and grounded. You have to question everything, examine it closely, and look at it from all angles negatively. Then everything will be fine. After all, you'd think you're prepared for anything.

However, it seems we give too little thought to thinking itself. For me, there's definitely a connection between thoughts, feelings, and health, and that's enough for me. At the top of my list for Mia's recovery options, therefore, is consciously positive thinking.

But I don't stop there. Therefore, I continue to research what our brain is capable of, even when damage has already occurred. I come across an article from a globally recognized medical research institute about "synaptic plasticity." I'm eager to find out if the brain can regenerate damaged areas.

If one part of the command center stops functioning correctly, can another part take over its duties? This question intrigues me. Because in MS, multiple inflammations typically occur in various parts of the brain, leading to dysfunction in the affected nerves. The nerve pathways can barely, if at all, transmit the corresponding nerve impulses.

This is why I need to know if other areas in Mia's brain can take over these currently disrupted functions.

And the institute's article gives me hope. According to neuroscientists, new nerve connections can constantly form. For instance, if nerve cells in the brain die due to a disease, neighboring brain areas can assume the roles of the affected regions. However, they can only do so partially, the article states.

But even partial recovery is enough, I conclude. If these nerve connections in the brain can be newly formed, then Mia should be able to walk again.

They even suggest that previous scientific evidence might be outdated, which claimed that nerve cells could only regenerate in the peripheral nervous system. Until now, it was believed that nerve cells could only form anew outside the brain and spinal cord. In the brain and spinal cord, this was thought to be impossible.

Now, they're not so sure about this anymore, I read, and it's a true relief. Because the spinal cord also plays a crucial role in the story of MS because inflammation occurs there too. And I am fully aware of what happens in this process. The myelin sheath, the protective layer around the nerve pathways, gets damaged, leaving the nerves partially or entirely exposed. It's like a cable without insulation. This exposure prevents the nerve pathways from functioning correctly. Now, neuroscientists believe that nerves can also regenerate in the spinal cord.

Additionally, there's the issue with the proteins that make up the damaged protective layer around the nerve fibers, which can normally heal. However, with MS, a specific protein in the body prevents the renewal of this protective layer. This means the myelin sheath can't be restored in MS patients.

Who really knows, I think at this point. Scientific knowledge is not static. It evolves constantly. And if the body can form new nerve connections and grow new nerve cells, then anything is possible. That's why I decide not to read lengthy, in-depth scientific studies that I would barely understand just to convince myself of the body's capabilities. I am satisfied with some understandable approaches that are backed by science and clear to me.

So, I delve into learning about the placebo effect, which I find highly relevant to the body's self-healing powers. Ultimately, I aim to shed light on all aspects of self-healing and offer Mia a convincing recovery plan.

If what I aim to present to her after my research isn't credible, then neither positive thinking nor any other training approaches make sense. We need facts. Things we can hold onto. As non-fictional as possible. Tangible and feasible. At least for us. So we can regain control of our life's path.

That's why I'm now reading about the placebo effect. This involves pills containing no active ingredients yet still having an effect. It includes surgeries that were never performed yet alleviate symptoms and why that happens.

The primary factor here is positive expectation and previous experience that patients have regarding a treatment or medication. This positive expectancy changes the neurochemistry in the patient's brain, leading to an improvement in health without the aid of medication or other treatment.

Numerous studies confirm this effect, I read, emphasizing the importance that the patient believes in the effectiveness of the medication or treatment. Recent estimates suggest that up to eighty percent of a medication's effectiveness may be attributed to the power of thoughts, which I find remarkable.

So what happens when patients take a pill to alleviate their suffering and the placebo effect is expected to occur? Just the thought of the healing power of this pill triggers the body to produce the same chemical substances that this pill would have produced. It essentially mimics the effect of this medication.

As I continue reading, I discover that prior experience with a medication plays a significant role in this process. If it has helped in the past, the patient is conditioned to believe it will continue to help in the future. This triggers the body's own substances, contributing to the placebo effect. The pill works without having directly cured anything.

Once again, I'm reminded of the importance of our belief in something for us to achieve our goals.

But what else lies in the labyrinth of self-treatment options, I wonder. I want to explore every possibility. That's why I delve into a topic I came across some time ago. In a TV documentary about athletes, they discussed how merely imagining movements can lead to changes in muscles.

I find this concept fascinating, especially considering its potential significance for Mia in her current state. Unable to move herself, Mia is limited to passive exercises with her arms and legs, which I perform for her.

However, I want her to feel like she's doing something. Visualizing movements could prove beneficial in this situation. But it only makes sense to me if they actually produce results. And for that, I need evidence. Because without proof, I can't tout these exercises to Mia as promising.

So I read that neither the brain nor the body differentiate between internal and external processes. When we imagine something, the brain doesn't distinguish between imagination and actual experience. Reality and fiction are nearly indistinguishable in the emotional center. That means, if you simply imagine a movement, say, of the leg, the nervous system perceives that movement as real.

This act of imagining, known as visualization, has been shown in numerous neurological studies to help patients rebuild their muscles after an injury or illness. Through experiments with test groups, researchers found that simply thinking about a specific exercise could effectively rebuild a particular muscle. One group visualized exercises for this muscle three times a day for five weeks, while the other group did nothing. And sure enough, the visualizers successfully trained and built up the desired muscle. All through mental training alone.

And that's exactly what I wanted to know. It works. Hence, we will promptly begin employing this technique.

Likewise, I will intensify the techniques I had somewhat disregarded with Mia in the future. Foot reflexology, acupressure on specific points. Prior to the thrombosis, I routinely massaged her arms and legs to enhance circulation. Once I get the doctor's approval, I'll resume these practices.

Finally, there's a topic that's intriguing, albeit not entirely proven. Nonetheless, it can't hurt. Affirmations. Mantras. The daily internalization of motivational beliefs.

I'm now delving into how all this relates to energy, quantum physics, and the law of attraction, even though I already know quite a lot about it. Nikola Tesla and Albert Einstein are mentioned, which I find impressive. Essentially, the Law of Attraction revolves around the idea that each of our thoughts emits a certain energy into the universe. If the thought is positive, the law of attraction ensures that we receive positivity in return, in the form of experiences, feelings, and the like.

Thus, affirmations will definitely be part of Mia's recovery plan. I've read several books on the Law of Attraction and affirmations a while ago and use them daily.

"Everything is working out for our highest good."

"All is well in my world and out of this situation only good will come." These affirmations have been with me for some time now, and they truly help me, especially in hopeless situations, to feel hopeful and motivated.

In the fall of 2018, I began using one particular affirmation that I repeat every day: "My daughter Mia is a positive medical miracle." And I firmly believe in it. Very strongly. 100 percent.

Ultimately, we can't go wrong, I conclude my research for now. If only a percentage of all these techniques and exercises work, we've already achieved something. Each progress, after all, is a step forward. A step away from where we don't want to be. And that goal is worth taking action for. Starting today. Every day. Tireless.

Monday, January 21, 2019

Sometimes, they say, you have to let go to eventually get what you hope for. It's not about fixating too much on one potential solution, frozen in fear of when it will finally come. No overthinking, no searching for explanations on how and when it will come to us. How it ultimately happened, I cannot fathom. But my wishing, hoping, and trusting did pave a path for the hoped-for to reach us.

Just two days after the medical board's rejection, Doctor Harper calls me around noon. Mia will receive a donation of medication from the globally recognized pharmaceutical company that makes the OC drug, he explains, as always, briefly and concisely. He doesn't boast about it, but from his few words, I gather that he must have worked hard to secure this donation.

And I have to admit to myself in this moment that I misjudged him and his humanity.

Thursday, January 24, 2019

Once again, it will be just a small, unremarkable vial containing something meant to have a profound effect, I think, as Tony, Mia, and I arrive at the Neurology Day Clinic on the morning of Thursday, January 24th. Once again, Tony had to carry Mia from the apartment to the car and lay her on the back seat. Because… well, because she can't even sit up without support. Once again, we transferred her from the car into a clinic wheelchair upon our arrival and have now reached the day clinic.

In my mind, there should be a fanfare at the entrance of the day clinic to welcome Mia. That's how significant this day is for us. The journey to this treatment has been so arduous. Yet, our arrival initially seems to go unnoticed by others.

We check in at the reception desk with the same lady who is always there. She tells me I can take Mia to treatment room 1. Tony is allowed to come along. Then we stand uncertainly in the doorway, and I look around for a nurse. "Oh, Mia's here," one nurse announces to the other nurses. They all know Mia. No one says anything as they see her in this condition. From their looks, you can almost hear them thinking, "Too late, this isn't going to work." Their faces clearly show the shocking realization of what this disease can do to a person.

Three years ago, they met Mia—a young, dynamic student who breezed through the day clinic with style. A few infusions and she was good to go again. Today, they see a different picture, one that is written all over their faces. But I choose to ignore that deliberately. Because I have my own prognosis for my Mia.

Shortly after, a young doctor explains that Doctor Harper has signed off on the treatment permit, and Mia can now receive the first infusion. Almost casually, she mentions how much Dr. Harper has advocated for Mia, after I express my relief over the long-awaited start of the therapy. He really took them on with the members of the medical board, she says. Yet they still said no, I think to myself. And now we've made it happen anyway. Without their approval. Thanks to his efforts.

I then ask the doctor if I could speak with him. "Absolutely," she replies, "he's in his office right now."

Doctor Harper is sitting at his desk when I enter the tiny office after a brief knock and his invitation to come in. He swivels in his chair to face me, meeting my gaze.

"Doctor Harper," I begin, pausing briefly. Of course, I've rehearsed a few lines in my head, but now that I'm standing before him, everything I could say seems inadequate.

"I don't know what to say. Because words can't express my gratitude. Mia... she's my only child," I try to explain, my voice choked with tears.

"I understand," he replies, and for the first time since I met Doctor Harper nearly three years ago, I see genuine compassion in his eyes.

"The medical board..." But he interrupts me.

"Those were unpleasant scenes, which I'll spare you from describing," he says.

In that moment, I realize that the Hippocratic Oath is not just an ancient physician's pledge for Doctor Harper. It's a calling to help his patients to the best of his ability and judgment, and to protect them from harm. Even when it seems hopeless.

He does this with few words, often misunderstood due to his reserved demeanor, which may appear as aloof and arrogant to many.

I almost feel ashamed because I've unwittingly painted a false picture of him. It's only now that I recognize his outward persona doesn't reflect his true nature.

He's a person and a doctor who is very much aware of his patients' suffering. One who doesn't say much but lets his actions speak for him.

Shortly after, I'm back in the treatment room where Mia is receiving her first infusion. Tony has stepped outside for a coffee. Meanwhile, I'm sitting on a chair next to Mia's bed. It must have been about forty-five minutes since the infusion started, and she's fallen asleep.

I glance around. Besides Mia, there are only a few patients in the large room today. Some are reading, dozing off, or quietly chatting with each other. Ultimately, time has to pass somehow. Once again, I realize that Mia is the youngest in this treatment room, and evidently the one with the most severe symptoms. Because no one here seems to be paralyzed in their arms and legs. They drink independently, walk to the toilet with the infusion stand alone, take off and put on their shoes without assistance. All the things my daughter can't do, I think, and it pains me.

At that moment, I recall the conversation I had earlier with a nurse while she was placing the IV access on Mia's arm.

She asked me how I was coping with the situation, like, for instance, washing her long hair. I explained that we had discovered our very own way of washing hair.

Of course, I didn't tell her how it was done. That Tony carries Mia and the urine bag into the bathroom, places her on a blanket on the floor by the bathtub, leans her back against the bathtub, then props her up with pillows on either side and holds onto her legs. So she doesn't tip over. This way, Mia can lean her head back slightly over the edge of the bathtub, and I quickly wash her hair.

I know, there are certainly more sophisticated options. But those aren't available to us in our bathroom. She can't fit into the large corner tub. We've already tried that. But she can't find a stable foothold in the wet tub, so she can't sit. So we opted for this somewhat adventurous washing maneuver. The primary goal was to get Mia's hair washed—that was our motto.

What the nurse said next made my breath catch for a moment.

"You could just cut her hair short. It'll be much easier. Just lying over a bowl. That works fine."

Even now, I find myself breathing hard as I replay the conversation in my head. How could she say that, I wonder, especially in front of Mia?

"Short hair is out of the question," I responded. "Mia's hair will stay as it is. Because she'll soon be washing it herself again," I emphasize, looking at Mia. "With a curling iron and all the fixings. That's what we're working towards after all."

And she'll be leaving the house on her own, I add silently in my thoughts. My prognosis allows for nothing less. Even after the latest MRI scans I remain resolute.

Shortly after the pharmaceutical company's approval, Doctor Harper ordered an MRI of Mia's brain. The scans taken just before starting the OC therapy are intended to visually document the treatment's success. I later read about numerous lesions in the report. In previous MRI reports, the exact number was listed, I noticed, and this vague description caught me off guard. "So it has come to this," I thought, "that they no longer count." Now they just write "numerous" and "significant". It made me realize what truly goes on inside her brain, hidden from plain sight. But it's good that we don't have to face the inner workings every day. It helps us focus on moving forward. And our journey continues here at the day clinic. The first step has been taken with the first infusion, I think now, looking at Mia as she still sleeps.

As euphoric as she was with the first medication, I noticed last night that she no longer feels that way. We were lying in bed together, talking in the dark, as we often do.

"I don't know if I believe in it anymore," she said. "Before the first therapy, I thought I'd have six or seven years of peace from the disease. And now. You can see for yourself."

I was relieved that in the protective darkness of the bedroom, she couldn't see my face, where the sadness about her condition was surely visible.

"Luckily, we still have other options. We're not dependent on this one medication. Just look at what's available and what the body can do on its own. The important thing is that we keep trying. We have to give it a shot. Otherwise, we'll never know if it could have worked. Don't worry, sweetie, we'll get rid of it," I said in a rush of words.

Just on Sunday, I had shared my newly discovered self-healing techniques with Mia, bit by bit. She was lying on the couch in the living room, and I was squeezed in next to her. I explained to her passionately that anything was possible if we just worked hard and stayed committed. Nothing happens overnight. But even with positive thinking, there's an immediate and noticeable effect. A sense of well-being and confidence that drives us forward. Especially her. And my enthusiasm for these newfound possibilities seemed to catch on with her.

"Oh, Mom, you're the best motivator," she said with a smile. "With you, anything feels possible and worth believing in."

And that's how it should be. Even though I can't be inside her head, I can certainly motivate her. I can help shift her focus to something positive during our conversations. Something that will hopefully keep her thoughts in a positive state for a few minutes, maybe even half an hour afterward.

"Come on, close your eyes," I urge her. "Imagine yourself walking. Where do you want to walk?"

"Through the forest," she replies with her eyes closed.

"What does it smell like there? What do you see?" I ask deliberately, so the image in her mind becomes as real as possible.

"It rained, and it smells like moss and wood. I see the sun shining through the tall tree canopies."

"Do you hear anything?"

"I hear the rustling of leaves and the snapping of twigs under my feet."

Leaves, I think to myself and smile. She loves the fall. That's why she thinks of leaves.

"Enjoy your walk, sweetie. Take a deep breath of the air. It smells of damp leaves and tree bark. You can still sense the freshness of the rain. Imagine how lightly you walk through this beautiful forest, letting the sun's rays warm your face. Here and there, you hear the crackling of branches underfoot and birds chirping in the distance. Somewhere in the treetops, you hear an owl. And you walk and walk. You feel every step. Your legs are light as a feather. And you walk and walk, happily and relaxed, through your forest."

– Chapter 12 –

February 2019

"That lady doing physical therapy doesn't need to come anymore," I declare somewhat irritably to Tony one morning in mid-February as we sit at the breakfast table, drinking coffee. "It's always the same. First, she shows up late because her cigarette break is apparently never long enough. Then, she drags out the session with unnecessary chit-chat. Finally, she does one or two passive exercises with Mia and says, 'Sweetie, you must be exhausted. Let's continue next time.' She's getting canceled. Typical insurance physical therapy…" I finish my rant and set my coffee cup down.

Initially, I had planned for Mia's physical therapy to start as soon as possible after her first treatment. Since I had always paid our physical therapist Ethan privately, I thought I'd combine his sessions with those from an insurance-covered therapist. Mia was entitled to it, so why not use it? I reasoned. Twice a week with Ethan, twice with the insurance therapist. And the remaining days Mia and I would handle on our own. I'd record every exercise on my phone, ask detailed questions, and then later guide Mia myself. That's how we'd been doing it for years, and it worked well.

But now we had Deborah, who appeared quite unmotivated. Before that, I had a nice introductory conversation with her on the phone. I explained Mia's current condition and our goals. "Yes, of course, we'll get it done," she said enthusiastically. She claimed to have extensive experience with such patients and excellent success rates. Well then, I thought. What could possibly go wrong?

However, as soon as the first physical therapy session ended—feeling more like a twenty-minute speed run—I realized it wasn't going to work out with her. Nevertheless, I wanted to give her a chance to prove herself next time. Unfortunately, the next two appointments went the same way.

"That's it," I decided immediately after the last physical therapy session. "You don't need to practice with her anymore, Mia."

"Well, thank goodness," she replied with a smile. "All that quick arm and leg shuffling isn't getting me anywhere."

So, I decide to have Ethan come only two or three times a week and manage the rest myself. Besides, anyway, Ethan can't come more often due to his work in a physiotherapy practice. And it's not feasible for my budget, I must admit. Especially considering other costs, of which I was already aware. Physical therapy marks just the beginning. I'll buy Mia a home exercise bike when she's ready. And other equipment she needs for her exercises. Even though she can't move her legs at the moment, I'm planning ahead.

After all, I've noticed that she's been using her hands better for a few days. She is able to take a pillow and throw it. Not always in the desired direction and distance, but we laugh about it and celebrate every little positive change.

Because, in my opinion, that's a huge step forward.

I try to remind myself of that over and over again. We need to shift our focus to the positive aspects. So my anger towards the physical therapist quickly dissipates.

"She's probably doing her best. But for us, that's just not sufficient," I realize, sensing how this mindset feels entirely different. No accusations, no bitter reproaches. That's the direction we're steering our thoughts toward from now on, as I had decided. Why keep complaining about everything? So, we're focusing our thoughts forward. Leaving behind what doesn't serve us.

And for the past two weeks, Mia and I have been starting our day like this. With positive thoughts. I've even compiled 'The Ultimate 11-Point Recovery Plan' for Mia in a PDF, which will keep reminding us of what we'll focus on in the future. In each of the 11 points, I've written in detail about what to focus on and what each point is intended to bring us:

1. Gratitude ritual
2. Positive thinking
3. Visualization
4. Affirmations (motivational statements)
5. Acupressure (to stimulate specific points on her body associated with symptoms like fatigue, pain, and muscle spasms, offering relief)
6. Massages (to alleviate muscle stiffness, reduce pain, improve circulation, and promote relaxation)
7. Foot reflexology massage (to stimulate nerve pathways, improve circulation, balance Qi flow, and promote relaxation)
8. Imaginary body exercises
9. Nutrition (anti-inflammatory diet, low sugar, limited animal products, reduced salt, essential vitamins, healthy fats)
10. Physical therapy (with Ethan, self-directed)
11. Trust in God

At the top of this list is the newly established morning gratitude ritual. Our day is meant to start with a pleasant feeling, even before I get out of bed and Tony carries Mia to the couch.

"Name three things you're grateful for. They can be seemingly insignificant," I begin.

"For the first rays of sun, for the soft bed, and for my mother."

"Not the same things every time, Mia," I say with a smile. "You can skip your mother."

"No, no. My mother has to be included every time," she replies, also smiling.

"And how does that gratitude feel? For the sunlight, for example?" I inquire.

"Nice," she starts, and I look at her. She smiles with closed eyes. "I feel happy when it wakes me up in the morning, knowing the sun is shining."

Quickly, I redirect her attention to the next image, knowing what might come next. The sudden realization that she can't just jump out of bed to enjoy the sunlight outdoors.

"Try to imagine yourself sitting on a bench, relaxing. The sun shining on your face, just enjoying it," I say, painting the next picture in her mind.

After I've listed three things I'm grateful for as well, our daily routine can begin. It hasn't always been easy to stay on track with our new positive thinking routine over the past two weeks. Sometimes, our thoughts drift. In those moments, we're both reminded of how long the road ahead might be. Still, I stick to it. We have to do something. So, everything in my ultimate recovery plan PDF will be followed at our own pace and with our own resources. Come what may!

At the end of the day, before bed, I introduce the same ritual. It's a way to round off the day.

"What did you especially like about today, Mia?"

Often, she lists the small, seemingly insignificant moments. A joke the three of us laughed at. Or the scent of the bathwater when I wash her on the couch. Because it's not always the big, overwhelming events that make us happy and grateful. Often, it's the little things. You just have to notice them and learn to focus on these details to enjoy them. Every single day.

In our supportive self-therapy, we also use techniques that I had subconsciously applied before. One such technique is visualizing the beneficial processes happening in the body. Especially during the daily massages of her arms and legs, as well as our own physical therapy sessions. I paint a mental picture of what should be happening in her body during these activities. Of the nerve pathways reactivating. Of the blood flowing freely through her veins. Of all the cells regenerating that we visualize together. Of her moving her legs by herself. Without any help. Through her own strength.

"Imagine it, Mia. Imagine exactly how it feels!" I encourage her to paint these pictures in her mind as vividly as possible and to truly feel them. Because it's the feeling that's crucial. The body should no longer distinguish between reality and vision. Her daydream should give her body a sense of how it reality feels. As vividly as possible.

Mia says her physical therapy sessions with Ethan have become the highlights of her week.

"At least I get to see someone other than Tony and you," she jokes.

And I believe her. It's a welcome change and a great help at the same time. Of course, before the first session two weeks ago, I explained to Ethan over the phone how Mia was doing. The last time he saw her was early last year when she was doing great. I didn't want his expression at the door to give Mia any hint of how he might feel seeing her in her current state. After all, he could be shocked since he could be in the same position, facing the severe symptoms of MS. Being an MS patient himself, he lives with that constant fear, which might show on his face when he sees Mia.

However, my worries vanished quickly when he arrived for the first session.

Since Mia can only lie down at the moment, he immediately started with hip stretching exercises in his usual straightforward manner. Lying on her side, he guided her to pull one leg towards herself. I stood by with my phone, recording everything so we could replicate it later.

I've started recording Mia's progress with my phone camera a few days ago. At first, it felt a bit strange, as if I was taking away a piece of her dignity. But I hope one day we'll look back at these videos with a relieved smile, proud of how far we've come. So, I decided my doubts were unfounded and kept filming diligently.

"Next time, we'll try sitting up, Mia," Ethan concludes after two weeks. "In the meantime, you can do some light abdominal exercises while lying down."

"I will," Mia replies.

And she does, starting the very next day. I film her. She lies on the couch in her gray sweatshirt and pink sweatpants, with one of her favorite songs, "In My Blood" by Shawn Mendes, playing on her phone. The catheter tube discreetly extends from her sweatpants to the urine bag on the floor next to her. Watching her through my phone's lens, I feel moved. She diligently bends forward, doing her best with the abdominal exercises.

She's so brave, I think, fighting back tears. She's brave and never gives up. That's my Mia. That's who she is and who she'll always be. When she sets her mind on a goal, nothing can stop her from achieving it, no matter the obstacles. No distance too far. No mountain too high. No water too deep.

This perspective on life is also evident in her decision to refuse a wheelchair, she mentioned to me a few days ago. Not even for home. She says she doesn't need it. After all, she'll be walking on her own again soon. Absolutely, then we won't get one, I say, giving in to her determination.

That's how it's going to be!

March 2019

In the quiet moments early in the morning, while Mia still sleeps beside me, I have this time all to myself. Just for a brief moment, I bask in the first signs of spring, enjoying them in solitude. It's crucial for me to gather my thoughts for the day and find motivation. I listen to the birdsong coming through the bedroom window and watch as the morning sunbeams illuminate the image of the Virgin Mary on the opposite bedroom wall.

Tony and I brought this picture back from our trip to Italy over ten years ago, and as I reminisce, my memories come alive. I recall purchasing it in Venice from a quaint antique bookstore. As we wandered through the winding streets of Venice, I stumbled upon the antiquarian while scouting for new photo opportunities down some alley.

The proprietor, with his gray beard and straw hat, reminded me of an older Italian artist, painting scenes of those same enchanting Venetian alleys where tourists rarely tread. Yet I could also imagine him in the evenings, sipping red wine amid his treasures.

Inside the antiquarian, I was greeted by an unexpected sight. Amidst the countless colorful bookshelves stood a retired gondola, its interior filled with stacks upon stacks of books. Cats roamed freely, lending the bookstore an eccentric yet cozy charm. At one end, an open green archway offered a glimpse of the Grand Canal.

I explored, capturing the essence of this extraordinary place in photographs, when I noticed sacred painting replicas adorning the walls, available for purchase. This one, I had to have. The one of the Virgin Mary with Jesus in her arms. Raphael had painted this marvelous piece at the dawn of the 16th century, as I read on a small plaque beneath the painting.

This is exactly how I envision her, I think now as I did back then. The mother with her child. Flanked by green velvet curtains, she appears to hover as if on a celestial stage above the clouds. In this very painting, she embodies motherhood for me. Holding her child protectively in her arms. Dressed in her blue robe.

In such moments, early in the morning, alone with my thoughts and memories, I look at the Virgin Mary and ask her for help. No matter how or when it may come.

"Please help us, Holy Mary. You know best what we need. Please help us," I whisper to her. And it almost seems as if she smiles back at me. As if to say, "Be patient and trust. Help yourself, and help will come."

In February, Ethan and Mia began their first attempts at sitting on the couch, and now, in mid-March, we're reaching a new milestone. Standing. It feels like progress is happening rapidly. Suddenly, we're already at standing. And this pace especially motivates Mia.

"Remember when you had to prop me up with pillows just so I could sit at all?" she recalls during a physiotherapy session, laughing.

"And how pale you got. Almost passed out," I add.

"See, and today we're already moving full steam ahead with standing," Ethan explains.

"I can't believe we've come this far already," I reply, looking at Tony. "Just a while ago… nothing was happening at all. It's truly incredible."

Tony smiles, standing in the middle of the living room, watching Ethan and Mia. He wants to memorize the upcoming procedure very carefully so he can practice standing alone with Mia later. That's what we've agreed upon. Meanwhile, I sit in the armchair and watch as well. I actually wanted to record this scene with my phone. But I'm too excited. After all, this could be a milestone in Mia's rehabilitation. This moment is too important for me to experience through the camera lens.

Ethan then explains to Mia that everything must be done very controlled. Mia is sitting on the couch, legs on the floor. The urine bag for her catheter is in a bag that usually sits on the floor. However, the tube leading from the bladder to the bag isn't long enough for standing. The catheter tube would come out. So, the bag has to go on the couch before they can start.

Ethan says that we should stand in front of Mia and reach under her armpits with outstretched arms. The outstretched arms should support her like two poles. Then she should slowly lean forward while sitting. Her legs should be at a right angle and hip-width apart on the ground. And then she should push herself up to standing with the strength of her legs and our assistance.

Just as I grasp what's happening, Mia is standing in front of Ethan. He continues to hold her. Like a dancing couple not dancing. A standing dance, so to speak.

"Phew, I didn't think standing would be such an effort," Mia says, beaming. "How tall you suddenly feel. The world looks so different from up here," she adds, and I can see the happiness over this unique moment on her face.

In this moment, I'm feeling like we're really making strides forward. Now that we've already achieved this, walking won't be far behind. Staying on track is crucial. It's essential that we stick to our mental and physical exercises every day. Then nothing is impossible.

In late March, Tony and I visit a medical supply store, often referred to as a "durable medical equipment (DME) supplier". Now that Mia's standing has improved, it's time to find her a walker for those first steps. With our assistance, she's managed a step or two already. But I want her to feel less reliant on us, and a walker can offer that independence.

Upon entering the compact shop and surveying the scene, I feel a sense of displacement wash over me. The walk through the store feels almost suffocating. Wheelchairs of various makes dot the space, alongside four or five different models of walkers on display. I notice the modest selection of adult diapers, bed pads, and such on the shelves. Moreover, I imagine it smells like sickness in here—like disinfectant mixed with a hint of mustiness.

In that moment, I can't help but feel like I don't belong here. Especially not with the task of purchasing items for my twenty-four-year-old daughter. How did it ever come to this?

But then, I force myself out of that dark reverie. Pull it together! After all, this is all about Mia's recovery. So, a walker is necessary for this leg of the journey. And a shower chair, too. With that, I'll be able to assist her during baths in our island home come May. Hopefully, we'll be able to make the trip in May, I think to myself.

That is, if the bladder catheter is finally removed by then. This thing has got to go. At the next appointment with the urologist, I'll push for an alternative to this indwelling catheter. The last attempt to remove the indwelling catheter a week ago was an utter failure.

Then I briefly recall our visit to the urologist last week, which still gives me stomach pains. The plan was to permanently get rid of the indwelling catheter. It was removed in the morning at the urological clinic's outpatient department. Afterward, Tony, Mia, and I were confined to the hospital grounds for the next two hours. In these two hours, Mia was supposed to drink one to two liters of water throughout the time to fill her bladder nicely.

So, we pushed her around the grounds in a wheelchair with a diaper on, and eventually settled into the nearby hospital café to while away the time. After the two hours had passed, we returned to the outpatient department, where they assessed how well Mia had managed to empty her bladder independently. But even at the café, I realized that it wouldn't work under pressure. Everyone knows the feeling when you can't use the bathroom under time constraints. Especially not in a situation like this. I had a sense that Mia's bladder would end up quite full, and the urologist would deem this attempt a failure. Well, that's precisely what happened. Indwelling catheter back in, appointment in two weeks, and farewell.

As I browse through the medical supply store looking for a suitable walker for Mia, I'm already planning how she can get rid of this bothersome thing. The urologist mentioned something about disposable urinary catheters that I could use to empty Mia's bladder several times a day. We'll take advantage of that, I decide, as I spot a walker that immediately catches my eye.

After about forty-five minutes, Tony and I leave the medical supply store with a top-quality walker and a bath seat. Both are sturdy and not nearly as ugly as I had anticipated, I joke in the car.

"What do you think, Nurse Betty?" I tease Tony.

Mia and I have been calling him by this nickname for a few days now. People say mothers don't get sick, but unfortunately, one morning, I couldn't adhere to this rule. Overnight, I had developed a fever of 102 degrees and felt utterly exhausted.

Damn, I thought, this can't be happening. How am I going to manage with Mia now? She still can't dress and undress herself. And then there's the diaper issue. I mentally listed all the tasks that needed to be done throughout the day. Tony could help her with eating, although she could already manage with her left hand. But what was I going to do about changing the urine bag if I wasn't able to? It needed to be replaced several times a day.

"I'll do it," Tony promptly volunteered. "It's no problem."

"Good, then today we'll call you Nurse Betty," Mia joked.

He really did his best, eagerly changing the urine bag. I explained the process to him in detail because, contrary to his assumption, it wasn't just about attaching and detaching the tube. The access to Mia's bladder catheter protruded from her sweatpants, and the urine bag's tube had to be connected to it. Unfortunately, there was a small catch that needed careful attention: if you didn't pinch the access with two fingers after detaching the tube from the urine bag, urine would start dripping out. On the other hand, you had to keep the tube of the full, detached urine bag elevated to prevent any spills.

The first bag change turned out to be a disaster. Mia and I were still in bed that morning during my feverish phase when Tony attempted his first try at changing the urine bag as Nurse Betty. Predictably, he forgot to hold the tube of the full bag up, and things went as they must. Urine spilled out of the full bag onto the parquet floor under the bed. We laughed until we cried. As we often did in such absurd situations.

Our bathtub escapades, for instance, regularly led us into fits of laughter. Because carrying Mia from the living room to the bathtub and bathing her was quite a meticulously planned endeavor. Alone with Mia in the living room, I first dressed her in a bikini. Then Tony carried her, with her urine bag in hand, through our small apartment hallway into the bathroom and placed her in the tub. Unfortunately, the urine bag tube would sometimes snag on something and come loose. And so, it happened that we would occasionally find a puddle of urine on the bathroom floor.

Mishaps that always gave us reason not to forget our humor even in such situations. Because humor was never lacking in our home.

April 2019

Finally, on April 15, it is accomplished. The bladder catheter has been removed.

"So, you're ready to empty Mia's bladder six or seven times a day using a disposable catheter?" the urologist asks me that afternoon.

"Yes, absolutely. Just show me how," I reply, not missing the undertone in her voice. It seems she believes the decision of when to remove the indwelling catheter should be hers alone. However, I've resisted that notion; we're prepared for the disposable catheters. I insist that a nurse just needs to teach me the technique of intermittent catheterization. It's time to free Mia from that annoying indwelling catheter. Besides, I believe she will soon be able to empty her bladder on her own.

The urologist narrows her eyes at me, skepticism clear in her gaze. Perhaps I've hurt her professional pride. But I don't care what she thinks about us, the catheter, or Mia's bladder; I have my own prognosis, as usual.

What concerns me right now is how we'll manage the catheterization during our trip to the island in May. I'm already picturing the difficulties. It's not like I can easily climb into the back seat at a rest stop to empty Mia's bladder in broad daylight. However, I won't dwell on that too much today, two or three weeks ahead of time. Let's see how it goes with her bladder, I reassure myself.

Maybe I've been worrying over nothing.

It was similar with walking. Back in January, I spent hours agonizing over how to get Mia back on her feet. And now, for the past few days, she's been taking a few steps with her walker from the living room to the kitchen and back. All by herself. So why all the constant worrying, I ask myself. Still, I'm glad we'll soon be heading to the island. In the solitude of our little fishing village, Mia can continue our recovery plan.

I also planned to buy her an exercise bike to improve her leg strength and muscle development. This way, we could walk a few steps around the house. With the walker. Or, more daringly, arm in arm. At least, that's what I envision as I put my plan into action at the end of April when the home bike I ordered online is delivered.

During Mia's MS-rehab last year in Maplewood, she told me about the workouts with the exercise bike. She would sit in a wheelchair directly behind the specially designed bike, allowing her to pedal from behind without needing to get up. Because sitting on the bike was impossible then, just as it is now.

I want to try the same setup at home, but without a wheelchair. Because she doesn't have one and doesn't want one. So, Tony and I place her in our living room chair, position the exercise bike in front of her facing backward, and assist her in placing her feet on the pedals.

But … the attempt fails. Despite how perfectly I had imagined everything, it doesn't work because Mia still can't control her feet. In my enthusiasm, I hadn't considered this. Her feet turn inward with her first tentative pedal, and I fear she might sprain her ankle.

"It's okay, sweetie," I try to comfort her when I see the first tears glistening in her eyes. Of course, she's disappointed. What did I expect? The bike arrives, and we're off on a Tour de Living Room?

"Everything takes time. We'll try again in a few days. Until then, we'll practice the foot-lift exercise Ethan mentioned. Okay?" I hug and hold her.

She nods bravely. But she wears her disappointment for the rest of the afternoon. And it's clear that my overzealousness is to blame. Slow down, I remind myself. Take it easy. We'll just take the bike to the island and continue practicing there, I decide later that night in bed and the thought soothes me a little. Despite the failed attempt. Because we must keep moving forward, I think, smiling.

– Chapter 13 –

May 2019

"You need to think about yourself sometimes. Why don't we go to a café or take a walk?"

"I just can't. As soon as I leave the house and think about Mia being stuck inside, I can't. It pulls me back home to her. That's just how it is."

"But she's in good hands while you're away. Just for an hour or two. On the weekend."

"I just can't."

And you don't understand, I add silently, remembering this conversation from two weeks ago at the end of May. I'm packing our suitcases in the bedroom for tomorrow's trip to the island.

I had this brief conversation with a friend I ran into at the nearby grocery store that day. She didn't understand how guilty I feel the moment I close the door behind me, step outside, and see the sun shining. When I smell the first blooms in the air and feel life happening outside. When I hear the cheerful laughter of children playing in the distance.

Then I know my place is with Mia. Until she can step outside and experience all of this again, I will wait.

There was no point in trying to explain this feeling to her, so I said goodbye and hurried to finish my shopping. I waved briefly. She wished us a pleasant trip and told me to get in touch when we got back. And then I was gone.

This conversation still lingers in my mind as I carefully pack Mia's clothes into her suitcase. Why don't others understand that I can't just leave the house? I am never truly alone. Thoughts of Mia and her situation are always with me. But what drives me is the belief that things will get better if we just keep at it. With our recovery plan. With positive thoughts, daily affirmations, all the exercises, physical therapy, and whatever else comes our way.

No one understands this, I think, while folding Mia's bikinis. I smile as I recall how happy Mia was with the new bikinis on May 13, her 25th birthday. Since she couldn't join me shopping, I went to the mall and got her three new bikinis. Of course, with a video call to make sure I got her style right.

I told her beforehand that even though it would spoil the surprise, it was important to get her input because returning bikinis can be tricky. Mia chose three styles to be ready for our upcoming island stay. Her bikinis from the last couple of years were too big now. She had lost weight after all the muscle loss.

But we'll fix that, I think now. The swimming exercises in the sea will help. They'll be part of our training plan once the water temperature allows it. By the end of June, it should be warm enough, weather permitting. Now that Mia no longer has an indwelling catheter, we have much more freedom in our planning.

About five days after the catheter was removed, Mia managed to partially empty her bladder on her own. Just as I predicted, I think, smiling. Now I only need to empty her bladder occasionally. This simplifies our daily routine immensely.

And we still need to sort out the trip to the island, though. But a solution will present itself, I think as I mentally review the steps of our journey tomorrow for the umpteenth time. What do I need to take with me? Where will we change her diapers? Can Mia get out of the car on the ferry, or should we stay in the car for the crossing? How do I manage the catheter situation? Everything needs to be sterile. Maybe we can make it without emptying her bladder. Mia suggested a few days ago that she could drink less during the four-hour drive to the ferry terminal. That way, we wouldn't need to empty her bladder at a rest stop. On the ferry, in the car deck, it would be more doable, I explained. When the other passengers are up in the lounge.

I hope I don't forget anything. The disposable gloves, disinfectant, single-use catheters, basin, and all the other items. While packing Tony's suitcase, I go over the list again and again. Then a thought hits me like a punch in the gut.

Grandma. She called the day before yesterday, I remember our last conversation. We had planned for her to join us on the island in a week or two. But she told me there was a change of plans, and suddenly, the line went quiet. She had a mild heart attack earlier this month and hadn't wanted to tell us. Even though she's much better now, her doctor has advised against any travel. Especially since it can get very hot on the island during the summer. The heat isn't good for her, the doctor had explained firmly. For a moment, I was speechless. I didn't expect this. It's not just the extra worry about my mother, but also her absence that weighs on me now.

You'll get through this, I try to motivate myself as I continue packing. You can handle this. You need to prepare the house. The garden. The vacation apartment upstairs. Our first guests are arriving at the beginning of June. I'll find out by the end of the season if I've taken on too much. With Mia, the house, and the guests.

Tony helps where he can, but he'll spend this summer at his parents' house. As usual. On one hand, all the work ahead frightens me. And then there's our recovery program, which carries so much hope and responsibility. Plus, I have my translation business to manage. If I hadn't had to cut back on my assignments so much in recent months, I could afford to skip renting out the vacation apartment this season. But I can't. Financially, that's just not an option.

So I constantly encourage myself. While packing our suitcases, doing housework, shopping, showering, and cooking. Over and over again.

"I can do this."

"Everything is always working out for me."

"I inhale positive energy with every breath."
"I love my life and life loves me."
And so on and so forth.

July 2019

"How would you evaluate the storyline?"

"Well, I must say, in the second third, it becomes quite tedious in some parts."

"I can only agree with you. And who do you think is the culprit?"

"I have a suspicion that Geraldine might have a plausible motive."

"You mean, to fully win the favor of her lover Peter, she got rid of his coheirs with a murder?"

"Yes, you might be right. Or perhaps… it was the gardener."

"Oh, Mia," I reply, laughing, "our book club is simply unbeatable."

Our daily reading afternoons on the terrace of our vacation house have become a cherished ritual. By six in the evening, the summer heat starts to wane, and we can sit outside in the gentle sea breeze. Each of us settles into her white rocking chair, the chirping of crickets providing a soothing background, and we begin.

I read aloud while she listens. We adopted this routine because Mia can't hold a book for long. We ordered the new thriller by our favorite author online, just like many other books. After all, the summer is long, and we won't let anything spoil our enjoyment of reading. Normally, each of us reads her own book.

But our situation calls for a new, yet old, way of reading—reading aloud. Initially, it felt strange to read a crime novel aloud to Mia. The dramatic reading of the novel's content was unfamiliar. It had been so long since the fairy tales of her childhood. But over time, I grew to enjoy it more and more, and now I give each character a unique voice.

This includes our pretend book critic, who also gets a fitting voice during our discussions about the current book. Overall, reading together is truly enjoyable. We ponder over the word choices, analyze the characters, search for the culprit, and question the psychological connections. Our daily reading afternoons on the terrace allow for all of this. They fill us with joy, curiosity, and enthusiasm.

Enthusiasm is something we've missed in recent months. It's an opportunity to genuinely take pleasure in something again. Like our beach visit last week. Mia could hardly wait to go swimming again. So, we set off for the beach. It wasn't as carefree as the summer before last, as this trip required a lot of planning. But in the end, our efforts paid off.

I had never really considered the obstacles a beach visit might present. Now, however, I was forced to think through every single step required to get us to our goal.

First, Tony and I figured out which beach would allow us to park the car closest to the water. We needed a beach where the parking spot was just a few meters from the water so that Mia wouldn't exhaust herself from the walk before she even had a chance to swim. Even with assistance, she would tire quickly after just a few steps. Thus, close parking was a must.

Next, we had to consider the beach's terrain. The small coves with sandy beaches were only accessible by boat, so that option was out, and I decided on a pebbly beach. On pebbles, Tony and I could support Mia as we guided her into the sea. However, she would need swimming shoes to make walking on the pebbles less painful. Because her walk was now different— more labored and less steady. Any misstep could make her lose her balance, and I wanted to prevent any discomfort or risk.

So far, so good. Park the car, walk a few steps to the beach with assistance, and then help her into the sea.

But what about the diaper? I had to think about that in advance. Changing clothes at the beach also posed a problem since we wouldn't find a secluded spot during the high season. So I planned for Mia to wear her bikini with an incontinence pad on the way to the beach. After swimming, we'd use a large towel to provide some privacy while she changed into a new pad. Once back in the car, she would put on a diaper again. Because unfortunately, she couldn't control her bladder; it would release when it needed to, often unexpectedly.

However, when the day finally arrived, things didn't go exactly as planned. How could I have anticipated how difficult it would be to navigate a pebbly beach and get into the water when you can't walk properly? Tony and I essentially hoisted her off the beach towel and supported her on either side. But the pebbles hurt her feet due to her uneven steps, and it took several attempts to make any progress. Walking into the sea wasn't possible, we quickly realized. Eventually, Mia just let herself fall into the water. And then… she swam.

"She's swimming, Tony," I exclaimed, thrilled. "She's swimming."

"It feels a bit strange," Mia replied from the water. "My butt won't stay under, but it's working," she said, laughing, and the joy on her face was unmistakable.

After swimming, Tony and I helped her out of the water, more or less dragging her along. "Like a limp seal," Mia joked, putting on her comedian face, which made me laugh even more. I asked her to stop joking so we could focus on our "seal rescue", but we could hardly stop laughing.

Ultimately, this first beach visit showed us that life can be fun in any situation, despite the challenges. Yes, there were sympathetic looks from other beachgoers, and yes, we felt like zoo animals being watched by a curious crowd. But we didn't let that bother us. What mattered most was how much we enjoyed ourselves and whether we achieved our goal. And we did. Mia went swimming.

August 2019

As early August dawns, Mia greets each morning around six with diligent physiotherapy exercises on the terrace. On her pink yoga mat, she stretches and lifts everything she can. She can do this alone now. And her walker is her constant companion. She does each exercise twenty times: squats on all fours, leg scissors, and ab workouts. And she keeps going like this for about an hour.

I admire her determination. No exercise is too hard for her because "no" is not in Mia's vocabulary. She has proven this time and again during her physiotherapy sessions with Ethan. Even in the toughest phases, she always wanted to try one more set.

Today, six months after her first attempts to sit up, it seems like a miracle to see how much she can do on her own. I tease her sometimes, joking that she's become a true aerobics pro. She then jokes back, "No one calls it aerobics anymore, Mom. Nowadays, it's just called a workout."

Of course, there are other days. The sad ones when Mia cries a lot. She then explains that the incredible effort she must exert daily to lead a normal life again weighs heavily on her. Nothing comes easy. She has to work hard for every new achievement. But it's worth it, I encourage her.

"Look how far you've come in such a short time."

"Yeah, I know. But sometimes I've just had enough. Constantly training just to walk a few more steps. Why can't I just live like I used to?"

And unfortunately, I have a hunch about what's causing these occasional mood swings.

"Stop looking at those pictures, Mia. They won't help," I try to address the root cause. She has once again looked at the glossy, joy-filled photos her friends post daily on social media. There are evening parties on the island, she then explains to me. Parties she can no longer attend. Who knows when that will be possible again, she adds. And she wonders how much longer this whole recovery will take. Sometimes, she's just tired of it all.

"No one expects you to be highly motivated and grinning widely while doing your exercises every day. It's normal to have down days. But then you have to keep going, Mia. We have a goal in mind. We can't do it without you."

"I know. Most of the time, I'm motivated. But sometimes, I'm just fed up with everything. It's hard to always think positively."

"It's not about always putting a positive spin on everything, Mia. The art of positive thinking is about looking forward again after the struggle and anger about your fate. Not burying yourself in self-pity. You don't always have to see through rose-colored glasses. But we can't stay stuck in sadness. Talk about it, and we'll figure out how to make the best of it. How to turn the negative into positive."

These are the moments we must overcome time and again to keep moving forward. To find the strength to reach our goal together. And in these moments, visualization helps us. An imaginary glimpse into the future that brings our vision of walking, jumping, and dancing to life on the screen of our mind's eye. Vivid and lifelike. In color and HD. A special visual spectacle where we are the audience. To get a taste of what's possible and let our bodies feel it. Simply through our imagination. And after five or ten minutes of such visualization exercises, things are better again. The courage is rediscovered, and the anticipation of what's to come is reignited.

These days, what also contributes to the constant uplift of our spirits is: the music. Something that ignites a love for a shared passion in both of us. So, we listen to the international hit list over and over again. No matter what's playing on the radio, we like every song, Mia and I have decided. With that in mind, I ordered a speaker online for us. We can even take it to the garden when Mia keeps me company there during gardening. We've named our speaker "Cindy," Cindy, our versatile talent. And Cindy can do it all. She can sing in all pitches, we joke. She's always spot-on with the lyrics, and Cindy has become an indispensable part of our daily routine. Even when Cindy's not singing, she keeps us entertained with stand-up comedy.

Lately, we've also discovered this for ourselves. Mia has compiled a proper playlist of our current favorite comedy stars for us to listen to over and over again. Every day, any time. Even in the early hours of the morning, if we feel like it and can't or don't want to sleep. Thanks to Cindy, we sometimes end up in James Corden's karaoke taxi until the early hours of the morning, singing along with him and the stars in the taxi. Since the beginning of July, our vacation apartment has mostly been occupied by guests. Consequently, we only allow 'loud' or 'very loud' music when the apartment is not rented out. Because even though singing loudly is much more fun, our guests have paid for the "quiet" spot in the midst of nature. Therefore, we must adhere to that.

Overall, I try to maintain a distance from the guests this summer. Even though I know they enjoy talking to me as a host about this and that, I keep mostly away. Mia doesn't want to be seen by them in this condition, and I respect that. That's why there must be a barrier. In recent years, it has occasionally happened that a guest came down to our apartment if they had a question or needed something.

"Do you happen to have a lemon squeezer? My wife loves freshly squeezed lemon juice for breakfast," for example. Or guests just felt like chatting. That has happened as well. However, this summer, I decide already in July when the first couple from Australia arrives, that's not going to happen.

"If you need anything or have a question, feel free to send me a text message. I'll come up or write to you."

That's the protocol, I add in my mind. After all, I don't want to risk a guest walking down to our apartment and encountering Mia in diapers and with a walker. That's something we must absolutely avoid, per Mia's request.

Only Tony and I are allowed to see her like that. Until, as she herself says, until she's the old Mia again. Hopefully soon, I think in those moments and try not to lose myself in the past. I try not to dwell on the past. Especially not about what could happen if things don't go back to how they were before. We're working on her recovery, I remind myself over and over. Working towards making it like it used to be.

Just as she desires. The life of a young, cheerful student who rushes out of the house in the morning to catch the bus to university on time.

– Chapter 14 –

August 12, 2019

"You don't need to be afraid; nowadays, there are medications that can manage the illness well. However, you should know that it progresses in your body, even when you're feeling fine and don't notice any symptoms," the doctor explains.

Well, I can't help but think, couldn't she lower her voice a bit? It would really set a more positive tone for the day, especially for the other patients in the room. Why doctors never tell you about what you can do yourself, I wonder. It's always about how well this or that medication works. Or rather, could work. Because no one can promise you anything. And they don't necessarily want to give you hope either. It's always just a 'probably' or 'presumably'.

These are all vague claims that no one can really understand and that can never be used against the doctors later. "But, you said…" That sentence doesn't exist because they don't allow it. No promises are made. Only a small glimpse of potential improvement may emerge from their patient discussions. I've understood that for a long time.

And it's the same with this patient, who is being informed about her new, faithful companion, MS, by a doctor in the Neurological Day Clinic in mid-August. Mia is currently receiving her follow-up medication dose via infusion. As usual, she's lightly dozed off, and I'm seated in a chair beside her bed, inadvertently overhearing the doctor's words.

A sudden chill runs down my spine. Likely due to the air conditioning, cranked to the max because of the scorching temperatures outside. Coupled with the words just uttered.

Because to my ears they sound like 'Have fun with the illness,' and the conversation's essence seems clear: 'There's little we can do to help.'

I discreetly glance towards the patient in question, sitting at the opposite end of the spacious patient room, apparently clutching a small stack of her reports in her lap. She gazes at the doctor, seemingly failing to grasp the meaning of what she's heard. It must be the shock, I think as I observe her expression. It'll probably take a few days for it all to sink in for her. Until she grasps it. Next time, and the time after that, she'll be sitting here with a growing stack of her reports, becoming a little more indifferent each time. Bit by bit, she'll get used to the fact that this has become part of her life. Whether she wants it to or not.

Perhaps she'll grow bolder, more energetic each time, because she's getting better at handling it all. Because she's symptom-free and feeling well. And because she feels safe. Because the illness isn't as bad for her as initially feared. She'll think she can live with that. Eventually, the terror of this diagnosis will fade. It'll become a memory that seems foolish in hindsight. Because she worried too much. Until the day she wakes up and realizes with a start that she is not alone. Her faithful companion has returned. Hidden in a symptom. A brief numbness in her arm, a heavy leg, or a momentary double vision in her left eye.

I want to get up, walk over to her, and encourage her. I want to tell her that she doesn't have to wait and see what happens or doesn't happen. That besides medications, there are techniques she can apply herself. After all, there's much more self-healing in our brains, our cells, our entire bodies than she believes.

I want to talk about visualization and what positive thinking alone can trigger in her. About what daydreams can achieve in our body. The neurotransmitters they release in her body and what that means for the proteins in her cells. How she should remind her arms and legs every day through exercises of how to move. And that she can mentally support every process in her tendons, bones, and every single cell positively.

Acupressure and massages are also very helpful, I want to say. I want to recommend daily affirmations to her. Statements to accompany her through the day and tune her subconscious to a positive outcome. Because our thoughts determine our feelings. And our feelings determine our well-being, I want to remind her. Which, in turn, has a positive or negative effect on our health. It's up to us alone, I want to emphasize. She has control over that. She can let the medications do their job and simultaneously contribute to her health.

With all of these techniques, she can motivate herself day by day. To look ahead when things aren't going well. Especially in those moments when everything seems hopeless. Just look, I want to say, my daughter is walking a few steps again. No one really expected that here, I'll add. Even the doctor earlier was very surprised to see her back on her feet after only six and a half months. I want to tell her how astonished he repeatedly looked at Mia and then her patient file. As if something didn't add up. He found it remarkable, truly remarkable.

But he didn't seem to attribute it solely to the medication, I inferred from his surprise. How did she do it, he seemed to want to ask instead. And in such a short time.

September 2019

"Eleven lines today," Mia announces one afternoon in early September, triumphantly raising a crutch to the cloudless sky. "Eleven times ten meters isn't bad at all, and I'm planning to add two more lines tomorrow. I always want to get better," she explains eagerly.

For about two weeks now, she's been practicing walking with crutches in a section of our garden paved with stone slabs. Cindy, our speaker, is always in the background, blasting Mia's training songs on repeat. Once again, "In My Blood" by Shawn Mendes fills the air. Meanwhile, I sit on a chair beside her, watching and filming her with my phone. It touches me to see how happy she is with every little bit of progress. Every line, every meter counts, she emphasizes repeatedly.

Seeing her now, my heart swells with emotion, and my mind drifts back to February, when she lay on the couch, immobile, in diapers, and with an indwelling catheter. I remember her first abdominal exercises when she couldn't move her legs yet but still began her training. To that same song. Always with a smile on her face, radiating her tireless zest for life.

She doesn't even wear diapers anymore, I think to myself now. Recently, she decided one evening that it was time to get rid of them. Incontinence pads from the drugstore will now do the job, she decided. Despite the occasional mishap at night. She doesn't care. The main thing is, they're no longer part of her daily life. She tossed them aside and moved on, just like everything else she's left behind and no longer needs.

When I see her now in the garden without those jogging pants bulging at the back, I understand what she meant about the freedom she gains from it. Even the disposable catheters, which I still occasionally insert for her when we leave the house, don't bother her. For beach visits or for half-hour rides around the island with Tony. So Mia can see something different for a change.

Later, when we move from the garden into the house, I think, we'll watch the video clips from February and today together. Then I'll show her the comparison between before and after. So she can see what she's achieving here and how far she's come already.

I'll even tell her that she won't need the walker much longer. At the moment, she only uses it at the end of the day when she's already tired and moving around the house. The rest of the time, she's started maneuvering within the house by lightly leaning on walls, doors, and furniture. She's learning not to rely entirely on the walker to support her body weight, but rather to gradually get her legs—and especially her core—accustomed to bearing her entire body weight.

At first, it was a bit challenging. In the first few days, she complained about lower back pain in the evenings. Ethan then explained to me over the phone which back exercises we should focus on. Her core needs to be systematically strengthened. Mia immediately incorporated these specific exercises into her training plan.

Ethan also said she should walk straight, he texted me later. Straight back, head up, looking forward. Yes, she's good at looking forward, I wanted to reply, but I didn't. I just smiled.

Just like now, here in the garden. I smile and rejoice with her over every line, every meter, every little moment of happiness in her recovery. And I record everything with my phone. So we can always make a comparison.

"You see, this is what it looked like just a month ago," I say. "And now you can already stand on one leg with support. Imagine what you'll be able to do in three or four months," I add, seeing the pride in her eyes.

Another two weeks pass, and it's September 17th. One day before my forty-sixth birthday. Mia and I enjoy the afternoon sun in our rocking chairs on the terrace. I brewed us fresh tea, and we discuss our latest mystery novel. Suddenly, Mia gets up to fetch something from the kitchen or so, she says.

But then, I watch—it feels like slow motion—as she rises from the rocking chair, briefly leans on it and then lets go. Before my eyes, she takes one step after another, walking five or six meters to the other end of the terrace. Without any walking aids. Without support. Without fear.

Instead, she's finally free, no longer trapped in her own body. Light as a feather. As if nothing had ever happened between the long-gone yesterday and today. As if there were no gap in time. In that brief moment, I see the Mia from a year and four months ago. A carefree young woman, walking here on the terrace of our house. Just walking.

And when I see the glow on her face, I feel that this is one of the happiest moments of my life.

We've finally made it. Mia is walking.

November 2019

In the fall, the city usually shows its most splendid side. It resembles a charming gentleman inviting us for an afternoon walk in the shade of the avenues. There, where the fallen leaves on the streets smell wonderfully of nature's vitality. Where little squirrels scurry about, collecting chestnuts from the ground and quickly climbing into the treetops. Along the streets lined with countless small cafés, where the still mild autumn temperatures allow for a brief outdoor visit. Wrapped in our fall coats, but with the cozy warmth of the autumn sun on our faces.

You'd think life is good here. Here, the city breathes its natural side. This year is no different.

That's why Mia and I set out for a little walk to a café. Linking arms, we walked the ten-minute stretch from home and now sit on the terrace of our favorite café with two cappuccinos.

"Just like old times," I say, squinting into the autumn sun.

"True. Almost," Mia replies, and I know what she is silently adding. A list of all the unspoken things that are no longer the same as before. "But it is really nice to sit here again," she then adds, knowing that we both are having part of this conversation in silence. Without needing words.

"The thing with college is weighing on you. I know. Just remember, it's not going anywhere. You'll get back to your studies. With a fresh burst of energy."

She falls silent for a while, and I let her be. The certainty that she couldn't continue her studies this year either is too painful for her.

We went through every conceivable possibility. How Tony could drive her to university in the morning and pick her up in the afternoon. That it would be no problem at all, and she shouldn't worry about the walks and the bus ride.

But then we tried to imagine the five or six hours during lectures in detail. The prolonged sitting, which she can't handle at the moment. She gets back pain after just an hour. And then there's her left leg, which she can't keep in one position for too long because of the thrombosis she had in January. She'd need to elevate it. I suggested putting it on a nearby chair, though it seemed foolish even as I said it. "How would that work?" Mia rightly pointed out. And then there's the issue with her bladder, she added. The restrooms aren't within reach. Not for her. How would she get there in time if she needed to go urgently? Incontinence pads, after all, don't offer unlimited protection.

I suggested that I could accompany her. I could wait in the hallway and help her to the restroom when needed. Be there if she required assistance. Five or six hours. I could bring my laptop and work in the meantime.

In the end, we remembered writing. Something so banal. Somehow, we had completely overlooked this point. "How am I supposed to take notes during the lecture?" she asked suddenly. I just looked at her. She could write again, but very slowly and illegibly. I suggested I could take the notes for her. "Somehow, all of this is possible," I said. Yet, I didn't want to make this decision for Mia. And so, she decided herself that it was still too soon. She needed more time. For her continued recovery. To be able to take the bus to university on her own, to walk better, to write better, and to be ready for university life.

So I applied for another year of leave for Mia with Mrs. Angel. I personally drove to the university, explained the situation to her in her office, and handed her the signed application. With tears in my eyes that I could barely conceal. "Mia has come so far already," I explained. "Just a little more, and she'll be ready for this too. For the daily routine, the many people around her. The rush, the stress." "I understand that," she replied, handing me an envelope for Mia.

Now, as Mia and I sit silently on the sun terrace of our favorite café, I think about Mrs. Angel's envelope for Mia. A greeting card. Both sides filled with tight lines. At the beginning a beautiful Bible verse and then words that explained what strength Mia proved. "You're a role model to be measured against," Mrs. Angel wrote. "What confidence and faith such a young person must carry within to master this great task of life. A task you tackle with aplomb, never losing your zest for life."

Her words still move me now, and I blink away a tear so Mia doesn't see what I'm thinking about as we drink our coffee. That's how she's always been, I think the next moment and smile. My Mia. Always determined, no matter what. That's the only way she manages to bear all this and still see the light at the end of the tunnel. Through her unique mindset.

Barely half an hour later, Mia and I start our walk back home when I suddenly spot someone on the street. I only know him from photos, but I recognize him immediately. He's standing about twenty yards away from us, waiting at a traffic light with his bike. He keeps looking around but hasn't noticed us yet. That must be him, I think, feeling my pulse quicken. I glance at Mia out of the corner of my eye as we walk, arms linked, in his direction. What do I do now? I wonder, my heart pounding harder.

I hope she doesn't see him. I need to prevent that. Turn green. Turn green already! I silently urge the light. If it turns green, he'll ride away before we reach the intersection.

"Maybe we could get another cappuccino tomorrow if you'd like. Then…" I try to distract her, keeping her gaze away from him as long as possible.

But before I can finish my sentence, it's too late. She has seen him.

She has seen Ben.

Just a faded shadow from her past, as she would describe him a few weeks later. Faded, to be forgotten.

– Chapter 15 –

2020

If I hadn't lived through 2020 myself, I would have thought it was the failed plot of a science fiction movie. The stage was the world, and we were the unwilling actors. In March of that year, an era began that would go down in human history, demanding much from us all.

A pandemic, practically overnight, became our constant companion. Without warning, it felt like a big bang had occurred, and suddenly, it was here. The virus. One that made us realize how fragile our existence on Earth really was. In the mirror of our existence, which was suddenly held up to us, we saw how tiny and insignificant we truly were. The virus spared no nation, age, or gender. It didn't distinguish between power, money, or influence. Fear crept into every home on the planet, that it might find its way there too.

This must be what the time after an apocalypse feels like, I often thought back then. Everyone fears everyone else. No one leaves the house without a face mask, and the fear that the virus could be transmitted through mere touch triggers a disinfection frenzy. A world in gray. People are standing in line for hours, desperate to secure the last rolls of toilet paper on their third attempt at the supermarket. Toilet paper, a commodity that seems as valuable as gold. Supplies are being hoarded. Uncertainty and fear of the future marked those seemingly endless weeks and months when suddenly, we were told to stay in our homes. Country borders were closed, isolating each nation from the others. To prevent the virus from crossing the barricades at the borders.

Until then, I had always thought preppers were crazy, with their delusional doomsday scenarios. Now, I watched their stockpiles of masks, disinfectants, protective suits, and food with envy on television. A treasure trove, with which they were obviously prepared for what was coming. How could this happen? In our so orderly world. Here in the city, the affluent society refuses to take even the smallest step backward. People are used to everything.

Living in the countryside seems more attractive than ever: self-sufficient, free, and independent. Tony and I started thinking about a greenhouse, a chicken coop, and fishing on the island. What it would be like, and if it was even possible. And this prospect of an alternative gave us hope. Nothing is lost. A life like that of our grandparents offers a long-forgotten sense of security, sheltered from the rest of the world.

Nevertheless, every time has its silver lining, I always say. So did March in the year 2020. It was meant to prove to me that my affirmation, "*My daughter Mia is a positive medical miracle*," had indeed come true. This affirmation had been with me for over a year now. Always in my mind and on my lips. Quietly, just for me, but always present.

No one knew it. It was my little, well-guarded secret. My affirmation that guided me until the day Doctor Harper asked me for the CD containing Mia's latest brain MRI scans. This time, the report stated "significantly less" and "much smaller". Finally, that day had come too, I thought, as I read the doctor's analysis of the MRI images in a report. Finally, the fruits of our efforts were evident there in black and white. The obvious and unexpected improvement in her health condition was now readable in these lines.

Doctor Harper was so amazed by this that he insisted on presenting these images at an international medical symposium, of which he was in charge. He wanted to showcase to his colleagues just how incredibly Mia's recovery had progressed.

And in his gaze, I saw the great astonishment at these facts as I personally handed him the CD. Of course, he didn't say what he was thinking: that he had never expected it in a million years. Such spectacular progress. From Mia needing nursing care to Mia walking. Even the most sophisticated medication seemed unable to achieve this alone, I concluded from his amazement.

She had done a lot for it, I explained, looking at him. Because she knew that medication alone wouldn't turn anyone from limping to walking. Instead, she had made her contribution to this success. Day in and day out, tirelessly.

That was in March 2020. In October of the same year, thanks to the introduction of online lectures at the university, Mia could finally resume her studies. From the comfort of home, she slowly readjusted to student life. The sudden slowdown of the world allowed her to catch up with the otherwise fast-moving pace of society, at her own speed.

And another year later, in October 2021, she could do things that seemed unreachable not too long ago.

She could snap her fingers, stand on one leg, tiptoe, write neatly, brush her teeth with her right hand, spoon soup with one hand, ride a bicycle, turn book pages, stand up alone from a squat, climb stairs, tie her hair in a ponytail, retrieve change from her wallet, pour a glass of water, tie her shoelaces, zip up her jacket, and walk independently.

And live independently.

Her never-ending drive has brought her to her goals. Through mental and physical training. Utilizing everything possible for recovery. From home exercise bikes, electrical therapy, and yoga mats to balance pads and hula hoops.

We conducted neuro-rehabilitation at home. Moving forward, backward, sideways, funny, funnier, wide-legged like a bear, nimble like a tightrope walker. Internet-guided lymphatic drainage was part of our routine. Massages, acupressure, and reflexology. We practiced positive thinking, morning gratitude, visualization, and affirmations. She trained, danced, practiced, thought, believed, and she walked, walked, and walked until she reached her goal.

We reached for the stars and grasped them.

Because dreams come true, you just have to learn the art of dreaming.

– Chapter 16 –

October 2021

"I love you, Mom. See you tonight."

She brushes a strand of her long, golden-brown hair from her face. On her left hand, the silver ring with the turquoise stone shimmers. The ring I bought her four years ago at a jewelry stand in Portobello Road, London.

"Love you too, sweetie. Have fun at university," I reply, giving her a quick hug.

As I close the door behind her, I linger in the hallway, closing my eyes and smiling as I breathe in the scent of her perfume. It carries the essence of her freedom, her young life, and the happiness in her eyes as she leaves the house …

Epilogue

Often, I look back and wonder how Mia would be today if she hadn't shown such unwavering determination. Amidst the many hardships and challenges she endured in her young life. Suddenly ripped from everyday life and catapulted into a place of seclusion from society. Where nobody asks what it's like to live in coexistence with the diagnosis of "Multiple Sclerosis". Unwanted and unasked for. With all her worries, concerns, and the pain of what was lost. Trapped in a body that no longer seemed to be hers. A body she sometimes believed she had lost control over. Yet in that place, she repeatedly found the courage and strength to rise above and defy the disease. Thanks to her inherent optimism, her belief in the extraordinary, and determination to achieve the impossible. Overcoming adversity and deliberately overlooking obstacles. Always looking ahead with her eyes to the sky.

In 2022, Mia successfully completed her Bachelor's in Public Relations. In 2024, she earned her Master of Business Communications Studies, attained certification as a court interpreter in three languages, and has written and published three children's books.

That's her. My daughter, Mia. A heroine whose bravery defies description.

For Mia:
My sweetie, never lose sight of your dreams, because …
Miracles are always just a heartbeat away.

Now that you finished reading this book,

it'd mean the world to me

if you left your honest thoughts about it

on your preferred retail platform.

Thank you!

About the author

Jasminka Vuković was born in Berlin in 1973 and is a professional translator fluent in German, English, French, and Croatian. Currently residing in a major city and an island with her daughter Mia and her partner, she divides her time between her work and her passion for writing. As the managing owner of her own translation agency, Jasminka enjoys crafting new book projects in her spare time.

Printed in Great Britain
by Amazon